SCRAWNY TO SWOLE

The Expert Guide for Men—Any Body Type, Any Age—To Gain Weight Fast and Get Ripped

REESE DOCKREY

Disclaimer

This book is for educational purposes only and is not intended to be a substitute for professional medical advice, diagnoses, or treatment. Talk to your doctor or other qualified health providers regarding any medical condition or before beginning a diet or fitness program. Not everyone who reads this book will get the same results; it depends heavily on the individual's unique factors and how strictly they follow the diet and training recommendations given.

For Mom

Contents

INTRODUCTION

Most people who work out want to lose weight; but you're not like most people. You're here to *gain* weight—healthy weight—and to get big and strong. That's what this book will teach you to do, the smart way.

Perhaps you're a young man who's been skinny your entire life, and you want to fill out your frame. Maybe even get jacked! Chances are you've already tried getting bigger and more muscular by eating more and working out, but it didn't stick. You probably have trouble gaining weight, even when you over-eat. The thought might have crossed your mind that you have bad genetics and that you're doomed to live in a scrawny body forever.

Or maybe you're a guy who has no problem putting on weight, but you'd like to change your physique. You're more "skinny-fat" than skinny, and you want to pack on some muscle without turning your little gut into a giant Santa belly in the process. But every time you've tried you just got a little bigger in all the wrong areas. You're curious about bulking up but also wondering if you should first do a "cut."

Perhaps you're an older man who's still underweight. Or you're at a normal weight with plenty of bodyfat but under-muscled. You've always been a little gangly and have probably assumed you'd be stuck with your unathletic body for life. You don't want to get fat but you do want to "fill out" a little, get more fit and perhaps pack on some serious muscle too. You want to know how to get bigger without simply ballooning out.

Maybe you're even an athlete who's spent years working out and eating healthy. You've packed on a little muscle over time, and you know the basics of general fitness. It's possible you used to be very muscular, but for whatever reason, you've lost a lot of "gains." You're ready to make a change in your diet and training that will get you more size and strength. Maybe you're inexperienced with bulking and training designed specifically to add lots of mass fast, and you want to know how to get started.

You're all facing a serious uphill battle. In order to gain not just weight but the right kind of weight, you have to build some muscle and not just add body fat, which you've likely never done to any great degree. You have to eat a lot and eat healthily, which you might not have much experience doing. You also have to learn (or re-learn) new workouts and maybe join a gym, both of which might seem intimidating.

Maybe you've searched online to learn how to do all these things, but the answers were confusing or it was simply too much information. One expert told you one thing, and another expert told you the opposite. I bet you even saw ads like this: "Get jacked in 30 days and lose fat at the same time!" Or, "Buy this supplement and you'll gain 20 pounds easily!" Unfortunately, that's all snake oil; a straight-up deception.

Here's Why Gaining (Healthy) Weight Is So Hard

"It's supposed to be hard. If it wasn't hard, everyone would do it. The hard... is what makes it great."
—Jimmy Dugan, A League of Their Own

The truth is, gaining healthy weight and building muscle is both *simple and hard*. It's simple because all you have to do is eat more of certain foods and do certain workouts. In fact, you could probably follow the advice of a basic one-page guide on "bulking" and gain lots of weight and muscle that way. However, if you want to bulk up the smart way and avoid the inevitable pitfalls of getting gains—unnecessary fat gain, wasted time in the gym, getting sick to your stomach with overeating, and so much more—you need to get more specific. It's hard because:

- The goal isn't just to gain weight, but to gain healthy weight. This means building muscle and avoiding unnecessary fat gains.
- You need to do specific workouts to build that muscle, or your extra calories will mostly just make you fat.

2

- You need to understand the basics of your unique physical traits so that you can eat and train accordingly.
- You need to know what foods to eat, how much to eat, how to over-eat with a tiny appetite, how to plan your meals, and how to afford it all.
- It's possible that bulking isn't right for you right now, and you need to understand your other options for gaining muscle and getting fit.
- The internet is full of confusing or even dishonest information about how to do it.
- It takes physical and mental discipline.

Transforming your body is difficult, much harder than simply dieting. In fact, that's why most people never even try. The good news is, if you're reading this, that proves you're willing to do the hard work! I know you can do it, because I did it.

"Dude, Who Even Are You and Why Should I Listen to You?!"

Simply put, I went from skinny to jacked in a year. Here's my story.

I grew up as a scrawny little kid. Despite having fast food and Dr. Pepper for every meal, I never gained much weight. The summer before my freshman year of high school, I lifted weights almost daily, but I got zero results. My buddies all hit growth spurts and began to fill out, while I still looked like the comical little brother on a Disney sitcom.

Being small killed my confidence and, while I hid it well, I was extremely self-conscious. I remember sometimes flexing my tiny biceps for hours at a time, just to make my puny arms appear bigger. Who I thought I was tricking, I don't know. I also avoided physical confrontation, and learned to make friends with the bigger guys early. For attracting girls, I relied almost entirely on my personality.

By the end of high school, I had finally hit my growth spurt and was now a foot taller, but I had only grown vertically. Now I was not only skinny but lanky too. I was a decent soccer player, but too weak and slow to truly be at the top of my game. I was more interested in football, but didn't even consider trying out, not even as a kicker. I felt completely unimposing and not respected by the other guys my age.

Well into my twenties, I could still eat whatever I wanted and my weight would barely fluctuate. It annoyed my friends that I could eat junk food without getting fat, while it annoyed me that they could get big arms with minimal effort in the gym. I had hoped that as I got older my body would finally "fill out," but it never happened. My metabolism didn't slow down a bit.

At the age of 28, I began a strict routine of bodyweight exercises at home five times per week. After a few years, I had gained a little more muscle but I was still very lean and nowhere even close to "jacked." The scrawny curse still wasn't broken. Even with all that working out, I would disappear when I turned to my side.

At age 32 (pictured right), I was 6'3 and 180 pounds. I was fairly strong and didn't look terrible, but I wasn't satisfied with being one of the "lucky" skinny people. I was sick of being small, and I knew I would have to do something different to finally change. One day I did a simple online search for "How to get big as a skinny guy." That's when I stumbled upon a YouTube series about combining weight training with eating big.

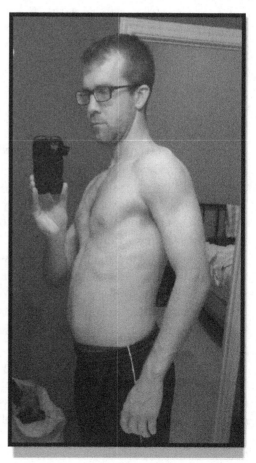

I didn't like the idea of eating lots of food, and I hated the idea of lifting weights. I didn't want to prove to myself how weak I really was, and I definitely didn't want to injure myself doing it. Losing my measly six-pack that I had built up by then didn't sound very appealing either. What I most dreaded was the idea of having to spend an entire afternoon online every time I had a question about what to eat, how to perform the lifts, etc. Still, I was motivated and I had the drive to put in the hard work. Turns out, that's all I needed.

I started eating the recommended stuff and lifting weights three times per week. I still didn't know exactly what I was doing, but I at least knew enough to get started safely. I was pounding protein shakes and putting peanut butter on everything. Having a physically demanding job on top of all this didn't deter me either. There were plenty of days when I didn't feel like eating more or working out, but it didn't matter; I had a mission.

The result? Within three months (pictured right) I had gained 30 pounds. It wasn't enough time to get absolutely jacked, but I was bigger, healthier, and I looked better. Within a year I had doubled my strength, too. Most importantly, I didn't get overly-fat or unhealthy in the process.

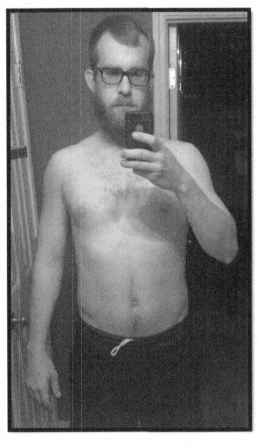

To achieve my goals, I still had a ways to go, and there was still a lot to learn. During those first few months, I got a lot of things wrong. You know how I gained 30 pounds in three months? Yeah, that was *way* too fast. Here are a few other things I got wrong, at first:

- I didn't follow a specific lifting program and sort of winged it the first couple of weeks, which failed big time.
- I went too heavy on some lifts (more than my knees are built for).
- I ate *too healthy* and too much bland food (e.g. chicken breast and spinach with no sauces).
- I ate gigantic meals, which made me feel sick.

- I didn't count my calories and ended up hitting weight-gain plateaus.

Still, I kept learning and making more progress. Eventually, I got it down, and I knew exactly what I was doing. On the right is a picture of me after roughly two more years of consistent weightlifting and on-and-off bulking.

Nothing crazy; I won't be winning any bodybuilding contests. But what's important is that this transformation represents essentially only two years of muscle gains (I missed out on several months of gains due to travel). And more importantly, I did it safely and naturally (no steroids), I did it all after age 30 as someone without special genetics, and it was all accomplished with a normal weightlifting routine (not a bodybuilding routine, which would produce even greater muscular size).

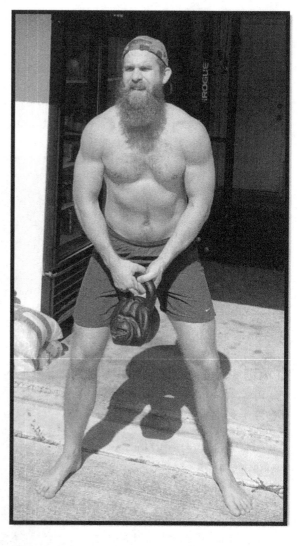

While researching how to get big, I discovered that the experts don't generally agree with each other about how to "bulk up" correctly. There was little agreement on how much to eat, which workouts were best, how folks with various body types should approach diet and training differently, and so much more. For a long time, I wasn't sure who to trust and whose advice I should ignore. Literally any claim I read by some fitness expert, there was someone else—also an expert—saying the exact opposite.

Others seemed more interested in selling their book or promoting their Instagram account than in telling the truth. Or, they simply didn't know what they were talking about. One author even claimed to have gained "10 pounds of muscle in a month!" No, bro, it's more like you gained four pounds of muscle and six pounds of fat and water weight.

I also noticed that experienced "gym bros" seemed to know more about the subject than most academics. Of course, it's not all the academics' fault. Most research on weight is about how to lose it, not gain it. After all, according to a 2016 report from the Centers for Disease Control, around 71% of U.S. adults age 20 and over are overweight, while only 1.5% are underweight.

Here's another key thing I noticed. While other books have been written about gaining weight, I found that they all seemed to target only certain groups—young people, super skinny people, people with only certain body types, and so on. But what if you don't know your body type? What happens if you're "skinny-fat" and you're wondering if you should eat like a super lean person? What if you're unsure if you still count as "young?"

More importantly, these other books generally don't explain your options or give alternative expert perspectives. Instead, they usually give a prescribed diet and workout plan which says "eat this much, follow this specific lifting routine," and so on. This is not a criticism of these authors, either. They understand that when it comes to diet and fitness, providing the reader with more of a one-size-fits-all approach makes things way less complicated. While some readers might prefer to be told exactly what to do, I prefer to learn about all of my options and make my own decisions. I also prefer to always get a second opinion (or third or fourth).

It became obvious that there wasn't a simple guide on "bulking" that cuts through all the online B.S., that applies to all men, and that incorporates alternative perspectives. So, I decided to do a whole lot more research and write the book myself.

I'm not a licensed dietician, doctor, personal trainer, or coach. Rather, those people were my teachers. I read countless articles written by university researchers, sports scientists, and world-renowned personal trainers and coaches. I also read the stories of hundreds of regular men trying to gain weight and build muscle. Their experiences painted a clear picture about what does and doesn't work.

Think of this book as one of those product-comparison charts you see on Amazon; you know, the ones where you can compare the pros and cons of various HDMI cables or whatever. In this book, I'll show you a comparison of the various diet and workout options you can try, and the results you can expect.

To be clear, this book isn't only for naturally skinny guys or just for beginners to strength training. It's for any man who wants to know how to add muscular size and strength, regardless of who you are or how you got to this point. Everyone who reads this will have a totally unique body and a history with diet and fitness specific to that individual. Whoever you are, the contents of this book will be enough to guide you to a quick and safe transformation.

I am not affiliated with any person, organization, or product referenced in this book. I'm not selling you anything; I'm just telling you what works.

Now, let's get started.

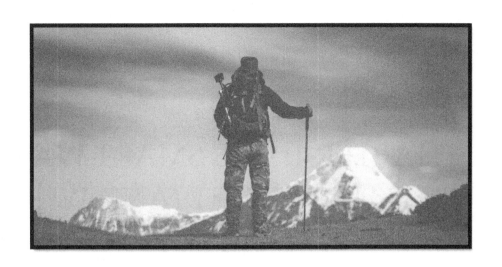

PART 1: KNOW THYSELF

CHAPTER 1: THE SMART WAY TO GAIN WEIGHT (AND WHY IT'S TRICKY)

"If you want something you've never had, you must be willing to do something you've never done."
—Thomas Jefferson

"Some people want it to happen, some wish it would happen, others make it happen."
—Michael Jordan

As you know, a human body needs a certain number of calories to be alive and active. Your body uses most calories to burn as fuel for everyday activities like walking, cleaning the house, taking out the trash, and automatic functions like blood circulation and breathing. To gain weight, you have to eat more calories than what your body is burning.

When you gain weight, it manifests as one of two things: body fat or lean body mass (LBM). LBM is the "good" stuff: muscle mass, organs, skin, tendon, ligaments, bone, and fluid. (Bowerman, n.d.) If you're generally inactive, calories that don't get immediately burned as fuel get stored as fat.

So, how do you store excess calories as muscle instead? In its simplest terms, building muscle requires overeating combined with working out.

The bad news is, when you gain weight to build muscle, some of your gains will be bodyfat. For most of us, there's no way around it. It's true that some people can gain a decent amount of muscle while burning fat, but that typically only happens when you have a lot of "fat stores" to expend, which you probably don't. In other words, generally only those who are obese can pull this off.

The exception to this rule, and the other group that can do this is steroid users, which I strongly recommend against. For everyone else, gaining muscle while simultaneously losing fat is a very slow process, and it can take years to see a significant change. Therefore, if you want a relatively quick body transformation, you're going to have to gain some bodyfat in the short-term.

The other bad news is, yes, you have to work out. I know, no one likes to hear that. *I get it.* I didn't want to either. The truth is, it's the only way you'll ever get the body you want. In order to generate more muscle tissue on your body, you have to work out.

The good news is, simply by eating right and working out regularly, you can turn most of those extra calories into muscle. You'll gain a little fat too, but you'll also be healthier and look better. You'll trade in your bony arms and six-pack (if you have one) for a thicker neck, bigger arms, more testosterone, and a thousand other desirable things. As a bonus, your body will get more of a V-shape, meaning wider shoulders and (the appearance of) a narrower waste. In fact, your waist might actually shrink, depending on where you start and which method you use to transform your body.

"Bulking" simply means overeating to gain weight while working out to build muscle. Bulking *the smart way* means doing all of the above while minimizing fat gain. First, you'll determine if a "cut" (losing weight while preserving muscle) or a "body recomposition" (gaining muscle while reducing your bodyfat percentage) are appropriate before bulking up. Then, ideally, you'll bulk and work out for a good while with potentially only minor changes to your schedule, anywhere from a few months to years. Then, to lose some of that new fat while keeping your new muscle, you restrict calories on a temporary cut or "recomp."

You can bulk, cut, and recomp as many times as you like, based on how you look and feel. Depending on things like your age and genetics, you might gain muscle very fast or relatively slowly. In the end, though, you'll be bigger, fitter, and leaner, no matter who you are.

3 Early Things to Know About Building Muscle

> "Exercise is king. Nutrition is queen. Put them together and you've got a kingdom."
> —Jack LaLanne

Later in this book, I'll go into much more detail about why and how to build muscle. For now, here are three initial things you should know:

1. Building muscle (usually) requires gaining weight and always requires working out. And not just any workout, but exercises known as "strength training." It involves moving heavy stuff around—things like barbells, dumbbells, tension cables, or your own bodyweight.
2. Strength training pushes your muscles out of their comfort zone and puts a great stress on your body. To recover from that stress and to repair your damaged muscles, you overeat and rest after each workout. This is the whole point of bulking, so that you can recover and bounce back bigger and stronger. (Kamb, 2020)
3. There's a limit to how much muscle a man can gain in his lifetime, and there's a limit to how quickly he can gain it. These limits will depend on several factors unique to each man.

A Few Myths to Get Out of The Way

In future chapters I'll be discussing the misperceptions of bulking and strength training in more detail. But for now, let's address the most common ones I hear all the time.

- *Some people just can't gain much weight.* This isn't true at all. If you've tried in the past and it didn't work, you weren't eating enough.
- *Some people can't gain muscle.* Not true. It's harder for some of us, but everyone can do it—any age or body type. If you've tried building muscle

in the past and it didn't work, the issue was with your diet, not following the right program (for you), or not following that program correctly.

- *Strength training makes you 'bulky.'* Actually, it burns more calories than most other types of exercise. It can shrink your waist and add weight to the areas where you want it. You'll only get truly massive if you're trying to.
- *To gain any muscle, you have to lift really heavy weights.* Nope. Moderate weights can do the job. The weight will be heavy *to you* and you'll certainly have to get much stronger than you are now, but you don't have to become an elite powerlifter.
- *To get fit, you have to work out every day.* Again, no. A couple hours per week is plenty.
- *You need tons of different supplements to optimize your training.* Nah. They might help but you don't need any of them to get gains. That is, muscle gains.
- *In order to eat healthy, you can only have boring stuff like rice, chicken breast, and broccoli.* Not even remotely true. You can have damn near anything you want, in moderation.

Chapter 1 Recap

To gain weight, you must eat more calories than your body burns. Your weight gain will be either bodyfat or lean body mass (including muscle). To gain muscle, you must strength train. This will mean adding some more bodyfat too. Bulking the smart way means gaining muscle while minimizing the fat gains. The whole point of bulking is to be able to recover from your workouts so that you build bigger and stronger muscles. There are a lot of myths about diet and fitness, but here's the truth: everyone can gain weight and muscle, you won't get huge unless you want to, you don't have to lift super heavy to get bigger, you don't have to work out every day, you don't need tons of supplements, and you can eat most things in moderation.

CHAPTER 2: DIFFERENT BULKS FOR DIFFERENT FOLKS

Everyone will have their own good reason for bulking up: to have a stronger presence, to be a better athlete, or simply to look good naked.

Everyone will also bulk differently. Not everyone should eat the same amount, or eat the same foods, or choose the same workouts.

In fact, if you ask an honest expert any question related to health or fitness, their answer will almost always be, "It depends." That's an annoying answer, but it's the truth.

What diet and workout routine are best for you? It depends on several things, including your age, workout history, personal goals, and more. Every choice has a trade-off, too. For example, one type of bulk will get you muscle gains more quickly, but it will result in greater fat gain. Another type of bulk will do the opposite; you'll gain less fat but it will take longer to achieve your desired body.

It's like buying a laptop. If you want the fastest one on the market, you'll have to get the big and heavy model. If you want the cool paper-thin model, it'll be slower. Point being, you can't have it all.

Ultimately, it's up to you to choose your own path. This chapter will help you choose wisely.

What Are Your Goals?

"Inaction breeds doubt and fear. Action breeds confidence and courage. If you want to conquer fear, do not sit home and think about it. Go out and get busy."
—Dale Carnegie

Before we get into how to bulk, it's important to first ask yourself, "What do I want to get out of my diet and training?"

I recommend actually writing these things down with pen and paper, or on your phone. It will only take a few minutes. You can do this now and then again after you've read the entire book (your goals might change by the end).

The *What*

Be specific and include a deadline. For example:

- "I want to add as much muscle as humanly possible in a year."
- "I want to double my strength and speed before next football season."
- "I want to be able to fill out that pair of shorts and t-shirt by next May."

The *Why*

Ask yourself, "Why do I have this goal? How will it benefit me? What bad things will I avoid if I achieve my goal?" For example:

- "If I fill out my frame and get more fit, I'll be more confident with my body and have a better chance with that girl I'm crushing on."
- "If I get more powerful, I'll be better able to protect myself and my family."
- "If I get stronger, I'll be more independent and won't need help moving my own furniture."
- "If I get more athletic, I'll finally have a chance at making the team."

The *Real*

Ask yourself, "How much time, energy, and resources am I willing to devote to eating healthy and working out?" Consider these factors:

- Only have time for a few 30-minute gym sessions per week? Choose an intense program to cram in the work in less time.
- Have lots of time but not much money? You can train at home for almost nothing.
- Have the money but don't want to join a gym? Build your own home gym.
- Want to bulk up but not willing to eat super healthy? If you're okay with more fat gain, you can still get bigger and stronger.
- Willing to eat healthy but not prepare the meals? No problem, as long as you can afford to eat out.
- Willing to eat only a little extra food and not a ton? That's okay, too! As long as you eat enough to build muscle, your gains will come slower but you can still get in amazing shape over time.

Now you know your goals, you know what will motivate you to do the hard work, and you know what you're willing to do to achieve it!

Your Unique Factors

Here's what makes your body unique: your body weight, body composition (lean mass vs. fat), genetics (muscle-building potential), age, fitness history, and body type (skeletal structure). Let's call these things your "unique factors."

Your unique factors determine which foods you should eat, how much you should eat, how you should work out, and the results you can expect.

How Much Should You Weigh?

First of all, if you're severely underweight, with a very low body mass index (BMI) or very low bodyfat percentage (BF%), you should see a doctor before starting any new exercise or diet routine. Whether you have a wasting disease like Crohn's or irregular eating habits like anorexia, you need to get to a safe weight. Being underweight can lead to all kinds of serious problems, including bone loss, decreased immune function, nutrient deficiency, and worse. (Battaglia, 2018)

Likewise, if you're overweight or obese, with a high BMI or BF%, you should also see a doctor before starting a new bulk. You shouldn't be gaining more weight until you talk with a medical professional about your current state.

Assuming you're not dangerously underweight or overweight, my suggestion is to initially focus on improving your body composition. That is, getting more muscle mass and ultimately logging a smaller BF% number.

Determine Your Body Mass Index

Your BMI is a simple ratio of your weight to your height. It tells you whether you're underweight, overweight, or somewhere in between. Luckily, it takes only a few seconds to determine.

I suggest doing so right this second. I personally prefer the Centers for Disease Control's BMI calculator (https://bit.ly/3kZkQyb), but there are many more free ones online, which you can find through a simple Google search on the subject. Nearly all of them will ask for your height and weight, while the more accurate ones will also ask for your waist circumference.

What Your BMI Tells You

The nicest thing about BMI is that a simple set of numbers apply to every person in every situation. Here's how those numbers break down:

- Below 18.5: You're underweight.
- 18.5-24.9: You're at a normal, healthy weight.
- 25-29.9: You're overweight.
- 30 and above: You're obese. (Assessing Your Weight, 2020)

Take note: just because you have a "normal" BMI, you're not necessarily healthy. You might still have too much body fat and not enough muscle mass. Also, you might be "overweight" but still healthy, especially if you already have lots of muscle mass. Such is the case with many elite athletes, and it's due to muscle being denser than fat. This is the drawback of BMI being so standardized, that it simply doesn't give you as accurate a look at your particular health. That's where BF% comes into the picture.

Calculate Your Body Fat Percentage

There are many different ways to determine your BF% number, depending on how accurate you want it to be and how much time and effort you're willing to spend. You can see a doctor or school medical center for the most thorough exam available. Or do it yourself with a skinfold caliper and measuring tape, which together cost ten bucks on Amazon. There are also "smart scales" that determine your BF% by sending a small electrical charge through your body, known as "Bioelectrical Impedance Analysis."

However, smart scales are notoriously inaccurate at determining BF%, calipers are difficult to use correctly without extensive training, and you might not have access to the expensive and time-consuming exam at a doctor's office. So my suggestion is to simply look at yourself in the mirror, then compare your body to what you see online. Do a search for "bodyfat comparisons" and you'll find websites with pictures of men compared at every BF% level. My favorite is at bodybuilder Marc Perry's BuiltLean.com.(https://bit.ly/3iRzYfh)

But be sure to find people who have similar muscularity to you. If you're a male with no muscle and a BF% of 10, you'll look nothing like the muscular athlete who also has a BF% of 10. For a great example of what I'm talking about, see this article by "Bony to Beastly." (bonytobeastly.com/skinny-guys-guide-body-fat-percentage/).

What Your BF% Tells You

Just as determining BF% is a more difficult process than determining your BMI, so too does it give a more accurate look at your body. The number ranges (for men) typically break down in the following ways:

- *Essential Fat: 4-6%.* It's "essential" because it's the bare minimum fat you need to survive. You need way more than this to be healthy, though. Don't forget that a certain amount of fat provides a very necessary function to your body—it protects your organs, maintains body temperature, produces needed hormones, and much more. Bodybuilders who get down to these BF levels experience all kinds of problems: lower testosterone production, higher anxiety and stress, and worse cardiovascular health than obese men. (Duquette, 2019)

- *Athlete: 7-10%.* This is considered healthy but still very low, potentially too low to build muscle. At this level, a man is still extremely "shredded," with a totally visible six-pack and high vascularity.
- *Fit: 11-16%.* Very healthy and the ideal range. Anything less than this might make you a better competitive athlete, but won't necessarily make you healthier. In fact, the health benefits of fat loss tend to end around 15 BF% and lower in men, but it differs with everyone. Some guys live very comfortably and healthily below this level.
- *Average: 17-25%.* This is where you start to look overweight. Probably too much body fat for the average person and perhaps starting to become unhealthy. However, plenty of fitness pros will allow their trainees to exceed 20% bodyfat, even if it's not "ideal." The numbers are not hard and fast, and there's wiggle room depending on the person.
- *Overweight/Obese: 26%+.* Very unhealthy. This is the range that leads to diabetes, hypertension, dementia, and a host of other medical problems. (Matthews, n.d.)

Chapter 2 Recap

Everyone needs to bulk differently, and it depends on your age, body type, goals, and workout history. It's up to you how fast you want to gain muscle and how much fat you're willing to gain in the process. You need to write down your specific goals, why you have them, and what you're realistically willing to do to get them. If you're at a healthy weight and bodyfat percent, you should focus on building muscle (you can drop the bodyfat later). Determine your Body Mass Index to know if you are at a healthy weight. It can be done online in seconds. Your bodyfat percent is easily determined by comparing yourself to pictures online.

CHAPTER 3: BODY TYPES AND OTHER FACTORS

Your Age

Being underweight is an issue for people of all ages, not just young folks. There's roughly the same number of people underweight in their forties and fifties as there are in their twenties and thirties. Same with those 60 and over. (Fryar, 2018)

Generally, the younger you are, the better you'll respond to diet and training. As you age, your body fat will naturally rise and your ability to build muscle will naturally decrease. I know, that's not great news. However, make no mistake, you can still transform your body, even after 40 and beyond. It just might take more time to get there, and more precision with your eating.

Gender

The simple fact is that there are numerous biological differences between the sexes when it comes to dieting and training. Here are the basics.

Men and women can work out in similar ways, but will have drastically different results. This is due mostly to the differences between testosterone and estrogen.

Males have 15 to 20 times the amount of testosterone as females. (Klepchukova, 2020) Testosterone is a key factor in body fat distribution, bone density, muscle growth capacity, and more. (Weatherspoon, 2019)

Put more basically, men tend to have more muscle and less fat than women, and can both gain more muscle and gain it faster. This means males can diet and train more aggressively. (Metabolism and Weight Loss: How you Burn Calories, 2017)

Genetics

Obviously, every person is born with equal dignity in this world. However, genetically speaking we simply aren't all born the same. Your potential gains depend heavily on things you can't change, including the size of your skeletal frame and your natural ability to build muscle.

For example, I have a buddy who lifts in his garage at home. The only lift he performs is the bench press, and he can lift over 400 pounds, despite eating a pretty typical American diet high in sugar and processed junk food. I don't know about you, but I can't do that. I lift at least three times per week, eat the right foods, and get my sleep, but I still have almost no chance of ever benching 400. I'm just not built for it. According to acclaimed strength coach Dan John, guys with long limbs and narrow shoulders—guys like me—generally can't get as strong as others. (John, Mass Made Simple: A Six-Week Journey into Bulking, 2020)

All body types can only get so big or so strong, or lose fat so quickly. This is called your "genetic potential." Some guys can barely touch a barbell and gain muscle like it's nothing. Others can spend years to get only a fraction of the gains. I can practice basketball every day for a decade and never be like Lebron James. That's because James' body is built for playing basketball. His genetic potential for strength and explosive power is leagues above mine.

It's not your job to become the strongest or biggest or leanest person ever. It's not even your job to compare yourself to your neighbor, co-worker or family member. Instead, it's your job to focus on becoming a better you. You might be surprised how much potential you have when you look at it that way!

Fitness History

"I was never a natural athlete, but I paid my dues in sweat and concentration, and took the time necessary to learn karate and became a world champion."
—Chuck Norris

Your experience with strength training (not just "exercise" in general) will have a big impact on how you should diet and train now. Training experience is usually broken down into three phases: beginner, intermediate, and advanced. With each jump to the next stage, the trainee is that much closer to reaching their full genetic potential for strength and size gains.

You're a beginner (aka "novice") when: you've never strength trained; or you used to train but haven't in years; or you do train but not with very challenging weights; or you've been training heavy but for less than six months. When you lift heavy as a beginner, you'll lack good form and you'll have no idea how the lifts are actually supposed to be performed. Your lifts will also feel shaky (literally) due to a weak nervous system. You also won't have a great sense of how strong you are yet or what weights will be challenging to you. You'll simply know what feels heavy *to you*.

As a beginner, you'll gain strength and muscle very quickly, and your training program can be very simple. Take advantage of it! By simple, I mean you can follow a program with only four or five lifts and short workouts (less than an hour) only two or three times per week. You'll experience "linear progression," meaning you should be able to lift a little more weight with each new workout. You might add 50 to 100 pounds to certain lifts in a matter of only a few months.

Of course, this rate of gains can't last forever. Generally, after six months to a year of consistently lifting heavy, you'll start hitting "plateaus" in the gym. This means your body is no longer responding to such a simple scheme of reps/sets and your body can no longer recover from your workouts as they are. Other things that will have improved dramatically: your muscular size, your lifting form, and your "mind-muscle connection" (i.e. certain lifts will just feel right to you while you'll notice a weakness with others).

Take note: It's important that you follow lifting programs designed specifically for you. So if you're a beginner, you shouldn't follow an intermediate routine. The fact is, some people remain beginners their entire lives despite working out with weights regularly. It's the price they pay for not following a program that's specifically designed to get them to progress from one stage to the next.

As far as bulking goes, since beginners can gain muscle the fastest, they can eat the most calories and bulk up more aggressively. As you become more experienced, you can't add muscle as quickly and should therefore use smaller and smaller caloric surpluses over time. A beginner who starts bulking with 800 extra calories might require only 100 extra calories after a few years.

Beyond the Beginner Phase

After this initial six months to a year, you'll hit the next stage of strength training: "intermediate." At this point, you'll need a new lifting program or at least make major adjustments to your current one, such as adding in more workout days, more exercise selection like isolation lifts and accessory work, and more volume in reps/sets. Your goals might change course here, too, and you might decide to pursue any number of training programs or athletics.

As an intermediate, your gains won't come nearly as quickly anymore, but you can still potentially add several pounds of muscle and 50+ pounds to your major lifts each year. If you continue bulking, you'll have to use a smaller surplus, and you might need to experiment with varied macro levels to find what works best for you (while always keeping protein high).

Generally, after two or three years of intense training as an intermediate, you'll progress to the last phase: "advanced." Although, it can take some guys a decade or more to reach this level. At this point, you're only able to add miniscule amounts of strength or muscle, and should therefore bulk with a tiny caloric surplus and expect very slow weight gain (perhaps a fraction of a pound per month). An advanced trainee is near their genetic potential, has probably battled some injuries as they reach their body's limits, and is likely lifting at least two times their bodyweight on squat and deadlift. This is an elite level of lifting, and just as most beginners never advance to become intermediates, most intermediates never become advanced.

If you're unsure what stage you're in, consider your current levels of strength and lifting skills. Ultimately, it all depends on how close you are to your genetic potential with each major muscle group. This should determine how you train and bulk, not necessarily how long you've been strength training or how big your muscles are. It's possible you've been lifting (or using a bodyweight program) for a decade, but if you haven't been eating enough or training correctly, then you haven't built a lot of strength or muscle. If so, you're still quite scrawny, and you're still a beginner. If you've been using lots of bodybuilder lifts like curls and you've gained some muscular size but you're still relatively weak overall, then you're still a beginner.

Perhaps you've been lifting for years and lifting relatively heavy, but your form still needs lots of work. If, for example, you can't squat to full depth, you can't deadlift from the floor with proper technique, or you can't bench press to your chest without shoulder pain. This means you likely haven't explored your full range of motion on the big lifts and therefore haven't maximized your potential for strength gains on those lifts yet. You're likely still a beginner.

It's also possible you're an intermediate on some lifts while a beginner on the rest, or advanced on some while intermediate on the rest. For example, I started lifting with a relatively high bench-press because I had been doing push-ups for years. Therefore, I was able to move my bench to an intermediate level quickly while my other lifts remained in the beginner phase for months longer. Meanwhile, my friend that benches 400 is advanced with his upper body lifts, but he's a beginner on the lower body lifts.

Your Body Type

This is your final factor in determining which diet and workout routine will work best for you. There are three main body types, and they are generic categories called "somatotypes." You almost certainly won't fit perfectly into any one category, and you're probably a mix of more than one. What separates each type is skeletal size (how large or small your frame is), how well you grow muscle, and how easily you gain fat. (Cortes, 2020)

You can do a search on this term to see images of all three somatotypes. I in particular like the one that can be found at MuscleAndStrength.com. (https://bit.ly/2Q6vRzB) I'll be referencing three types of bulks that correspond with these three body types— small, normal, and big. We'll look at these bulks in more detail in later chapters, but for now let's examine the three body types.

Ectomorphs

If this is you, you have a narrow skeletal frame and a thin bone structure. You also have very little muscle. It's likely that you're naturally skinny and also tall and lanky. Common features include long and thin limbs, a flat chest, drooping posture, and small wrists, shoulders, and neck. Many ectomorphs have a hyperfast metabolism and smaller stomach which make it difficult to gain weight. You probably eat like a bird and feel sick when you try to overeat.

The bad news first: Gaining weight (and therefore muscle) is usually going to be harder for you. That's why skinny guys are often called "hard-gainers." When you're a hardgainer (not all ectomorphs are), you have a harder time gaining weight due to a faster metabolism and a smaller appetite. This means you have a harder time overeating, and you have to eat more than others to gain size. Possibly *a lot* more (e.g. the "big bulk"). The fact that you might have a smaller stomach than average doesn't help either.

Thankfully, eating more will get easier for you over time. It's well established that stomach size can vary person-to-person. What's not as well know is that stomach size can adapt to dietary changes. When you overeat, your stomach expands temporarily, usually causing discomfort and bloating. However, when you consistently overeat, your stomach will expand more easily, causing less discomfort. (Chavoustie, 2018)

One cause of your unusually efficient metabolism is the fact that you expend lots of calories from what is called "nonexercise activity thermogenesis" (NEAT), which includes fidgeting, changing posture, and other basic, often subconscious activities. In 2000, Mayo Clinic researchers found that fidgeting can "substantively contribute to energy balance" (i.e. burn considerable calories), especially fidgeting while standing, such as adjusting your standing position. (Levine, 2000)

In fact, the researchers at fitness website Bony to Beastly (an excellent resource for hardgainers) reviewed the aforementioned study and found something incredible: Hardgainers burn 50% more calories from sitting than the average person, and 80% more when standing. They also estimated that a hardgainer can burn anywhere from 600 to 950 extra calories per day just from standing. (Duquette, 2020) If you're someone who's constantly standing, fidgeting, and generally moving around a lot, that's partly why you burn calories like a champ.

The last bit of bad news: As an ectomorph, you'll start off very weak. Your long, lanky arms and legs, your muscle-fiber composition, and your hormones can be a hindrance to your muscle gains. But make no mistake, *you can gain weight and put on tons of muscle*. It might just take you more effort. Focusing on eating a lot will be your top priority. To turn those extra calories into muscle, you'll need to lift heavy stuff, too.

Ectomorphs: Blessed, Not Cursed

The good news: To be clear, you're called a hardgainer only because you have a hard time gaining *weight*. It doesn't mean you have an especially hard time gaining *muscle*. Once you do start gaining weight, you can gain muscle like crazy. In fact, you can potentially gain muscle two to three times faster than others (I'll explain why in a later chapter). This should be music to your ears if you're a skinny guy who's tried lifting weights and didn't gain a thing. Now you know, it's not that you can't build muscle, or that you're a "non-responder" who got the short end of the genetic stick, it's that you almost certainly weren't eating enough.

Other advantages to being an ectomorph: as you likely have greater insulin sensitivity, you're better at building muscle; your awesome calorie-burning abilities also mean you'll gain less fat than others as you build muscle; you'll retain your awesome ability to burn fat after building lots of muscle, so maintaining a low bodyfat percentage and looking shredded year-round will be easier. In a way, *you have the best body type of all.*

Mesomorphs

This is the athletic body type. If this is you, you likely have a normal body weight and appear lean (15% bodyfat or less) and muscular, with well-defined arms, broad shoulders, good posture, and more of a rectangular shape. Mesomorphs are born with "lucky genes" and are more likely to naturally excel in sports. They gain muscle (but also fat) easily.

If you are naturally athletic and a beginner to training, you might do best with a "normal bulk," since you can gain muscle efficiently. If you're an intermediate, you can't gain muscle as quickly anymore and should consider a "small bulk." If you're happy with your body but would like to slowly add more muscle and get even leaner, you can do a "recomp." (i.e. gain muscle while dropping your bodyfat percentage) while eating maintenance calories. You can also add more cardio than an ectomorph can.

Endomorphs

Endomorphs have a high natural BF%. Other features include a round physique, thick limbs, short stature, and a slow metabolism. They tend to gain muscle and fat easily. A higher insulin resistance means they easily store excess calories as fat. They also have more natural muscle than skinny people, especially in the lower body, due partly to carrying around more weight. They'll likely excel at lower body movements like squats.

If this is you, you shouldn't bulk at all. Your best option is to cut or do a recomp while on maintenance calories. If you want to lose weight and get to a healthier bodyfat level quickly, do a cut. Being overweight and a beginner to strength training means you can gain muscle while actually losing weight (not just clocking a lower bodyfat percentage) on a cut. If you're not a beginner, then you have lots of muscle already, and you'll look great after a cut or slow recomp. Once you're back to a healthy bodyfat level, you can bulk up with a "small bulk." Anything more than that might be too many calories, as you will retain your ability to rapidly put on bodyfat as you bulk.

"Skinny-Fat"

This fourth category is an in-between type, very common and easy to define. Basically, if this is you, you're at a normal weight but your BF% is too high, and your body likely appears overweight due to extra stomach fat. Your main issue isn't your high bodyfat, it's that you're simply under-muscled. You have no shape due to your lack of muscle; it's just bones and bodyfat. Ectomorphs also lack muscle, but due to their extra height and lower body fat, they don't appear flabby like you do.

Being at a normal weight while having too much bodyfat is extremely common, too. In fact, 29% of men have a normal BMI yet are at an increased risk of developing diabetes and heart issues due to their low levels of muscle and high levels of bodyfat. (Duquette, 2019)

Making your appearance worse is the fact that you probably have bad posture, too. People with little muscle mass tend to tilt their pelvis forward which pushes their stomach out, making it appear as a bigger gut than it really is.

You might have been very skinny when you were younger, and later in life developed some extra weight around the midsection, through a combination of aging, poor diet, and a lack of muscle-building. Or maybe you have a healthy diet and do intense exercise like running or even a moderate version of CrossFit, yet neither of these things seem to be affecting the shape of your body. Either way, you aren't building significant muscle, so most of your extra calories just get stored as belly fat.

This also means, like ectomorphs, you are almost certainly a beginner. If you were an intermediate, you'd have more muscle, and you wouldn't have such skinny limbs.

(For a great starting place to learn more about the skinny-fat type, I recommend this science-based article from the sports supplement supplier Legion Athletics [legionathletics.com/skinny-fat/]).

The Skinny-Fat Problem

The main problem for skinny-fat people is that to gain significant muscle, you need to gain weight, which means gaining more fat. But you already have a high BF%. So, what do you do?

We already know that when you do gain weight, it's mostly belly fat. When you lose weight, you don't look fit. Instead, you look like you're starving. Your dilemma is simple: you want to gain weight without looking fatter, and before gaining weight, you might want to lose fat without looking weaker. Unfortunately, you can't have it all, and you'll have to make a trade-off.

How you should begin your transformation depends on how much bodyfat you currently have. If you're at an obese bodyfat level (over 25%), you can perform a cut until you're leaner, preferably below 15%. Beginners might even build significant muscle during this phase, and they will definitely get stronger. At the very least, you can preserve your current muscle. The downside to cutting is, if you don't build muscle, you'll end up looking even scrawnier as you lose weight. The upside is the cut might last only a few to several weeks, depending on how much fat you need to lose.

Your other option (if you start with over 25% BF) is to perform a "recomp" to slowly lose fat and potentially add a little muscle while maintaining your current weight. You'll never get weaker-looking like on a cut, but it will take longer, potentially a few months or more. Whether you cut or recomp, you'll eventually be lean enough that you can begin bulking for faster gains.

If you're currently between 15 and 25% BF, your bodyfat level isn't ideal, but it isn't as dire a situation as the 25%+ group. Cutting is also an option for you, but you'll likely prefer a recomp. It will still be a slow process, but it won't take as long since you aren't far from an acceptable bodyfat level. Once you're below 15% or so, you can then bulk up for faster gains. This will also give your body time to build strength. As you improve your diet with more protein and cleaner foods, your nutrition partitioning will also improve (i.e. your extra calories will finally go to building muscle instead of fat). If you can't wait that long, you can try a very small calorie surplus (such as the "small bulk" or even less). I'll discuss how to do all of these—bulking, cutting, and recomping—in later sections.

When you strength train, you skinny-fat guys will finally add weight to the areas where you want it: arms, legs, shoulders, upper back, and chest. During the recomp or cut phase, you'll lose the belly fat, too.

Similar to ectomorphs, skinny-fat guys have the potential to add a ton of muscle, since you don't have much to begin with. Once you get down to a healthy bodyfat level, you can start bulking for faster gains than your cut or recomp will allow. Since you'll still have the propensity to add fat easily, you'll need to use a more moderate bulk than hardgainers (no more than a "normal bulk."). That's unless you're more "skinny" than "skinny-fat." The harder it is for you to gain weight, the more you can bulk like a hardgainer.

Regardless of the body type you start with, after enough bulking and training (and perhaps a cut or recomp to start), you'll be lean and muscular.

But it all starts with the food. And what exactly should you be eating on a bulk? Let's finally tackle that in the next chapter.

Chapter 3 Recap

All ages struggle with being underweight, while younger guys will respond better to aggressive dieting and training. As a man, you're better equipped than women to build muscle and bulk up fast. How fast you can get big and strong is determined by your genetics as well. Regardless of your age or genetics, you have tons of potential. Beginners will see the fastest rate of muscle and strength gains, although after a few months the gains will continue but at a slower pace. As you get closer to your genetic potential, your diet and training will have to be adjusted accordingly.

There are a few main body types: Ectomorphs are skinny, usually tall, and typically have a harder time gaining weight; they can burn calories very well and their top priority is eating a lot. Mesomorphs have athletic bodies and don't have to eat as much to grow but can still eat and train very aggressively. Endomorphs are overweight or overly fat and shouldn't bulk. Skinny-fat people have too much bodyfat and not enough muscle; their best option is usually to recomp before bulking up slowly. All bulkers can cut or recomp whenever they want to, and they will eventually be bigger and leaner.

CHAPTER 4: CALORIES AND WHAT TO EAT

"Let food be thy medicine, and medicine be thy food."
—Hippocrates

Dietary considerations aside, calories are simple. Eat too much, you gain weight. Eat too little, you lose it, no matter if it's healthy food or junk food.

In 2010, a nutrition professor at Kansas State University proved this point. He lost 27 pounds in 10 weeks by eating 1,800 kcal (aka calories) per day on a diet of almost entirely Oreos, Doritos, and Twinkies. His point was simple: to lose weight, you just have to eat less calories than you burn. (Park, 2010) The same is true of gaining weight; just eat *more* than you burn.

Of course, you shouldn't actually get all your new weight gains from junk food. We'll look at this subject more later; but for now, let's examine the simpler issue of just calories themselves.

Caloric Surplus, Deficit, And Maintenance

Calories are energy stored in food. They're like fuel for your body. When you eat a meal, you give yourself a lot of energy in one sitting, like filling up your car's gas tank. Most of the fuel gets burned through automatic body functions: breathing, blood circulation, brain activity, support of vital organs, etc. Add up all of these calories and that's your "basal metabolic rate" (BRM). Simply put, your BRM tells you how much energy your body would need to lay on the couch all day and just exist.

The remaining calories burned in a day are fuel for digestion and physical activity like walking and exercise. The calories that don't get used throughout the day, your body stores as "future energy" in the form of fat or lean mass (including muscle).

When you add up every calorie you burn on an average day, that's your amount of "maintenance calories," also known as "Total Daily Energy Expenditure" (TDEE). You maintain your current weight with this amount. Men tend to burn about 2,500 to 3,000 kcal per day, but it varies. Generally, you burn more when you're taller, younger, more muscular, or more active. If you're shorter, older, or inactive, you require less.

Using the Baylor College of Medicine BMI calculator, let's quickly compare the same man at three different ages. He's very inactive and weighs 175lbs standing at 5'9 (the average American male height, according to the CDC). At 20 years old, he'll expend around 2,680 kcal per day. At 30, around 2,580 kcal. At 40, around 2,490. Now let's compare a man at three ages, but this time he weighs 200lbs at 6'0 tall, and he's very active (maybe an athlete or he has a physically demanding job). At age 20, he needs 4,070 kcal; age 30, 3,970 kcal; and age 40, 3,880 kcal. As you can see, the number of calories you require is heavily influenced by your age, size, and activity level.

When you eat maintenance calories, your body weight stays about the same week-to-week. If you under-eat one day, you're likely to over-eat the next day, without even thinking about it. On the other hand, long-term undereating or overeating requires some effort.

Let's say your maintenance calories are 3,000 per day. If you eat 3,500 kcal one day, then you have a "caloric surplus" of 500 for the day. If you eat only 2,500 kcal, then you have a "caloric deficit" of 500 for the day. This is your "energy balance," meaning the relationship between how much energy you give your body and how much it expends. A surplus means you're in a "positive energy balance," and deficit means you're in a "negative energy balance."

You've probably heard of the laws of thermodynamics. Well, the first law states that energy can neither be created or destroyed, instead energy can only be transformed from one form to another. With food-energy (i.e. calories), you give it to your body, and your body transforms that energy into fueling your daily activities or storing it as "future energy" to be tapped into later. All dieting to gain (or lose) weight follows this simple principle.

You can think of surpluses and deficits in terms of budgeting, if it helps. A budget surplus is when you save more money than you spend. So if you save $10 one day, that's a $10 surplus you keep in your wallet for future expenses. It's just like when you eat more energy than your body needs, and you can use that extra energy to "buy" some new muscle. Likewise, a budget deficit is when you spend more than you bring in, which is like burning more calories than you eat in a day.

Calculate Your Maintenance Calories

To figure out your maintenance calories, use pen and paper to track your food intake for a week. Eat and drink like you normally do and record every calorie—meals, snacks, drinks—using food labels. Or, do it all with an app like MyFitnessPal or MyPlate. Then, take that total and divide by 7 to get your daily maintenance calories. (Or if you're finding the process too tedious, simply counting your calories for three days will still give you a decent approximation.)

An even quicker (but less accurate) option is to calculate the number online for a rough estimate. There are several free ones, but each website uses a different formula, and the results vary wildly. The one I recommend—as it seems to give a sort of average of all of the various online calculators—is found at TDEEcalculator.net. Whichever site you use, most will ask for your gender, age, weight, height, and activity level. Some will also ask for your bodyfat percentage, but it's optional.

For the final (and least accurate) option, Harvard Medical School recommends a very simple method for moderately active people to estimate their maintenance calories. Simply multiply your bodyweight in pounds by 15. That's it.

This isn't surgery, so once you have your exact number of maintenance calories, feel free to round to the nearest whole number to make it easier to remember (e.g. 2,891 becomes 2,900). Whatever your TDEE is, then when you daily eat more than that number consistently, you'll gain weight. Consistently eat less than that number, you'll lose weight.

Working Out Will Increase Your Maintenance Calories

Assuming you don't currently workout regularly, then once you start strength training, your body will require higher maintenance calories. A 2004 Harvard Medical School study estimates the numbers like this:

- At 125 pounds, people will burn 180 kcal per hour of training.

- At 155 pounds, people will burn 224 kcal per hour of training.
- At 185 pounds, people will burn 266 kcal per hour of training.
- At 200 pounds, people will burn 310 kcal per hour of training or more.

Basically, once you start training hard (being defined here as around three hours a week of intense exercise), your maintenance calories will increase roughly 100 kcal per day. For example, if you weigh 185 pounds and you started with maintenance calories of 3,000 per day and now you train a few hours a week, your new maintenance calories are around 3,100 every day (including the days you don't work out). This is only an average, though, and you might burn more in less time. Of course, if you already train consistently, then your TDEE shouldn't change much.

Now you should know approximately how much energy your body expends daily. Later, I'll help you decide exactly how many extra calories to add to your diet to start bulking up, or how much to cut to start losing weight.

What to Eat

For the next few months or beyond, you're going to be eating a lot more than usual (if you're bulking). More importantly, you might be eating healthier stuff than you're used to. This brings many challenges, like knowing which foods to eat, how to factor in your own unique circumstances to know how "clean" you should eat, and understanding the pros and cons of less-than-healthy foods.

You've heard a thousand times that most Americans eat a pretty terrible diet, and it's true. We have way too much highly-processed carbs, added sugar, seed oils, and much more. If you eat lots of this stuff, you'll have to unlearn a lot of bad habits. You also might have heard some rumors about how healthy dieting is boring, tedious, expensive, and so on. As someone who grew up on fast food and then started eating right, I can tell you that those rumors are just dumb.

Let's nuke a few of those myths right now:

- *Your diet has to be really strict and your food choices are very limited.* Not true. You can still eat whatever you want, but in moderation.
- *Fat and cholesterol are bad for you.* Nope. Moderation is still important, but both are essential, and there are good and bad versions of each. They play a role in making hormones and vitamin D, building cells, and much more.

35

- *Eggs and dairy are bad for you.* This is a big misconception. Eggs alone have essential nutrients like zinc, iron, antioxidants, vitamin D, and brain-boosting chemicals like choline. (Gelman, 2020) Dairy also has tons of protein and there are plenty of options with less fat (such as substituting whole milk for 2%, or liquid egg whites for whole eggs).
- *You shouldn't eat more salt than food labels suggest.* A growing number of academics are disputing this. Plus, the more active you are, the more salt—a natural electrolyte—will benefit you.
- *Gluten is making you sick, bloated, and gassy.* Unless you have a specific gluten-allergy or celiac disease, then it's likely something else that's causing you to feel this way.
- *You have to buy "superfoods" like kale, chia seeds, kombucha, apple cider vinegar, and alkaline water.* This is a marketing gimmick. Sure, these things might all be good for you, but any natural food (without processing or additions) is a superfood.
- *Being healthy requires expensive "health food" and supplements.* Nah. I'll explain this in more detail later.
- *You have to buy fresh produce.* Actually, fresh fruit and vegetables often lose lots of natural enzymes during the shipping and storage process. Frozen and canned produce, on the other hand, preserves much of its nutrient content. (Gelman, 2020)
- *Carbs are the devil.* Carbs are essential for building muscle. Some people might need a moderate amount, but they aren't bad for you.
- *Low-fat and no-fat products are good for you.* Maybe, or maybe they just substituted a bunch of sugar for fat to make it taste good. These labels are often adverting tricks.
- *You'll become obsessed or even develop an eating disorder.* Your bulking or cutting diet won't last forever, and it's simply a tool to get you to your goals. You don't have to think about food all day or make it your identity.
- *Once you start a diet, you can never stop it, or you'll lose all of your progress.* Nope. Once you build some muscle from bulking, you can go on maintenance calories for years without losing any gains.

Whole Foods

"About eighty percent of the food on shelves of supermarkets today didn't exist 100 years ago."
—Larry McCleary, neurosurgeon and author

"Don't eat anything your great-great-great-grandmother wouldn't recognize as food."
—Michael Pollan, Harvard professor and author

Honestly, you already know what foods are good for you. It's "adult food." I'm talking oatmeal and fruit for breakfast instead of Captain Crunch.

The most important rule for eating healthy—eating like an adult—is focusing on "whole foods." These are foods that are as close to their natural form as possible. They're called "single ingredient foods" because they aren't combined with anything, and contain little to no processing.

Basically, anything that grows in the ground, on a tree, or on an animal is a whole food: vegetables, fruits, nuts, beans, and legumes. You can also include unprocessed meat, grains, seafood, and dairy. They're all high in nutrients with no "empty calories," and they're filled with the stuff your body needs for training, such as protein, healthy fats, complex carbs, fiber, vitamins, minerals, and phytochemicals.

This runs counter to the typical American diet which includes lots of preservative-filled packaged goods, highly-processed carbs, added sugar, seed oils, lab-produced "food," and much more. Since you might be unfamiliar with healthier food options, I've provided a few links below where you can learn more. I personally most enjoy the ones found at HealthLine (healthline.com/nutrition/50-super-healthy-foods) and BetterHumans (https://bit.ly/2Q3gI22).

Dirty Vs. Clean Bulking

"Eating crappy food isn't a reward — it's a punishment."
—Drew Carey

Simply put, whole foods are "clean," while "dirty" food is greasy fast food, processed sugary carbs, sodas, chips, pizza, etc. You've probably heard of "dirty bulking" (aka dream bulking), which means eating only the crappy stuff and none of the good stuff. It's a terrible idea for most people, and it's a common rookie mistake that a lot of guys make when they first get into muscle-building.

If you're super skinny and you hate over-eating, then you'll no doubt be tempted to load up on junk food. After all, eating half a pizza is a lot easier than eating a couple plates of rice and grilled chicken. The thing is, you can still eat some junk while maintaining a mostly healthy diet. We all love food that's bad for us and we all get emotional about what we eat. That's normal. I'm not about to tell you that you have to start eating like a robot. Still, if you're an average American, you probably need to eat healthier than you currently are.

It all comes down to smart choices. Have grilled fish instead of fried. Have a baked potato instead of French fries. Order the side of fruit instead of the side of mac and cheese. Snack on mixed nuts instead of chips. Have an omelet and black coffee instead of syrup-drenched French toast and whipped-cream-laden Starbucks "coffee" (which is the nutritional equivalent of a blended birthday cake). Drink water, tea and calorie-free soda, instead of full-sugar soda and glow-in-the-dark "sports drinks" (which often have more sugar than even soda).

"But wait," you might think, "if I'm going to be overeating and gaining weight, why does the quality of the food matter? I'll be gaining fat and muscle either way." True, but here's what a dirty bulk will do to you:

- You'll gain more of the wrong kind of fat (visceral fat located inside the abdomen), potentially leading to arterial plaque buildup.
- Your body won't get all the essential nutrients it needs to build muscle, so, you'll miss out on gains.
- You'll get an inferior mix of nutrients, which will make you tired, unmotivated to work out, and generally feel gross.
- Due to the thermic effect of food (TEF), you'll waste more energy on burning processed junk, making your workouts less efficient.
- An abundance of simple, processed carbs, like is found in chips, pizza dough and hamburger buns, will lead to more insulin resistance, which leads to a higher possibility of diabetes. (Evans, 2019)
- You'll very likely gain too much weight too fast, which means you'll gain way more bodyfat than you want.

- Your eventual "cut" (when you burn the fat you gained while bulking) will take way longer.

How Clean Do I Have to Eat?

> "So, when it comes to eating healthy, it's just doing the right thing. And it's not something you have to do 365 days a year, but I think it's something you have to do 25 days a month. Let's put it that way."
> —Mike Ditka

Like any other diet, you get out of bulking what you put into it. With a dirty bulk, you eat like crap, so you look like crap and feel like crap. The cleaner you eat, the better you'll look and feel.

However, *you don't have to eat a perfectly clean diet.* In fact, most trainees shouldn't even try a bulk of exclusively 100% whole food, because it's just too easy to fall off the wagon. Bulking is hard enough, so there's no reason to make it even harder by not giving yourself some meals to look forward to. Like most things in life, the key is in moderation.

How clean should it be? Let's say you shoot for a bulk that's 80% clean, 20% dirty. That's great! That means you get to enjoy a "cheat meal" one out of every five dinners. 90:10—even better. 70:30—still decent. 50:50...er, dirtier than I would recommend.

Also, you don't have to spread out those cheat meals evenly. You can eat totally clean all week, then have an entire "cheat day" on Saturday. Or, make every meal 80% healthy, so that you're having a "cheat ingredient" instead of an entire cheat meal. Or simply eat healthy throughout the day and then have dessert after dinner every night. There's no real wrong way to do this. Just find what works for you.

Consider Your Age and Body Type

As a general rule, the older you are and the easier it is for you to gain weight and body fat, the cleaner your diet should be. The 80% goal is still fitting.

If you're a tall, skinny person—i.e. an ectomorph—who has a very hard time gaining weight, you should still eat mostly clean. However, you need to make every calorie count. Even if it means eating a little dirtier than is ideal. You definitely shouldn't be filling up on vegetables and grilled chicken alone. You must focus on eating lots of calorie-dense foods (more on those later). In fact, you'll probably benefit from occasional cheeseburgers and pizza, too. They aren't clean, but they do have tons of calories and protein.

Add It in Pieces

I recommend taking a few weeks to add in these new healthy diet changes. For instance, if you want to eventually eat a clean-to-dirty ratio of 80:20, start on day one of your bulk at 60:40. The next week you can make it 70:30, and finally 80:20 on week three.

Don't stress over hitting these exact percentages. One day might be 90:10, the next day 65:35. Remember, this is an art, not a science. As long as you consistently eat a majority of your food from clean sources, you're on the right track.

Since suddenly eating lots of food and mostly healthy food can be a big challenge, you can always start a healthy diet before bulking. You can do this in parts as well. For example, you can start by cutting most sodas and sugar. A week or two later, cut most of your microwaved meals and replace them by cooking with whole foods. After that, replace processed grains with whole grains. And so on. These incremental changes will help you acclimate to a healthier diet, and give you more confidence that you can eventually start a bulk and stick to it.

Chapter 4 Recap

All you have to do to gain weight is overeat, but there's a right way and a wrong way to do it. First, you need to determine your maintenance calories which is how much you eat daily to maintain your current weight. Eating more than this requires effort and is called a caloric surplus; eating less is a caloric deficit. Track your food for up to a week to determine your maintenance calories, or use an online TDEE calculator for a less accurate estimate. Round the numbers to an easy-to-remember figure. Working out will increase your maintenance calories by around 100 per day.

You need to focus on eating whole foods which are natural, single-ingredient foods with little to no processing. This includes fruits, vegetables, nuts, beans, legumes, meats, grains, seafood, and dairy. Use the internet to find more healthy options. You need to eat mostly clean foods and not "dirty bulk" with mostly junk food. Try to always eat healthier options when available. Dirty bulking can help you build muscle but it can also have devastating consequences including gaining too much fat, gaining the wrong kind of fat, missing out on gains due to malnutrition, less energy, and higher risk of diabetes and arterial plaque buildup.

You don't have to eat perfectly clean; 80% clean is a common goal for bulkers. You can still have plenty of cheat meals or cheat days. Generally, older guys need to bulk even cleaner. Young hardgainers can get away with more junk food. Consider taking a few weeks to slowly make your diet healthier by introducing more clean foods.

CHAPTER 5: MACROS

All food can be broken into three categories known as macronutrients: protein, fat, and carbs. How you break down these three "macros" into percent of total calories is up to you.

It doesn't have to be over-complicated. As long as you're getting enough protein needed to build muscle, there's a ton of wiggle room for your fat and carbs. However, you still need both. Eating a very low-carb or very low-fat diet will make bulking and gaining muscle difficult if not impossible.

According to trainer Alexander J. A. Cortes, macros in percentages of total calories should be based on body type as follows:

- Ectomorphs/hard-gainers: 50-60% carbs, 20-30% protein, 20-30% fat.
- Mesomorphs: 30-40% carbs, 30-40% protein, 30% fat.
- Endomorphs: 20% carbs, 40% protein, 40% fat. (Cortes, 2020)

These are of course general guidelines. You don't have to hit these exact numbers. The best way to get your macros is through food, but pills and powders are also a good and safe choice. If you prefer to follow a specific food plan, "If It Fits Your Macros" (IIFYM.com) is a popular one. If you use it, make sure you get the necessary protein (and fiber) and still focus on mostly whole foods.

Protein

When it comes to building and maintaining muscle, protein is *by far* the most important macro. The Recommended Dietary Allowance for protein is 0.36 grams per pound of body weight (Pendick, 2015), but this is simply the minimum amount you need to function normally and not get sick. Adding muscle (and keeping it) requires way, way more.

Most diet and fitness experts agree that eating at least *1 gram of protein per pound of body weight* is both safe and sufficient for building muscle. Therefore, a 180-pound man would eat 180 grams of protein per day.

Tall hard-gainer men might need even more, up to 1.25 grams per pound. This might be more than necessary, but it's still safe. Plenty of experienced coaches and trainers recommend even greater amounts, especially for young men.

Likewise, maintaining muscle on a cut or recomp might require higher protein intake than one gram per pound, for everyone. If you ever eat more than your body actually needs, it's not a problem.

Oh, and in case you've heard that excess protein is toxic to your body, it's not. Any protein you consume that your body doesn't need will simply be excreted or used for fuel. Assuming you don't have an underlying condition, it's not going to poison your kidneys or turn into fat or whatever. (McKay, 2020) Even consuming 2 grams of protein per pound of bodyweight—twice the amount I recommend—wouldn't hurt you. (Schultz, n.d.)

Keep in mind, as your body weight goes up, so should your protein intake. If you gain 10 pounds, you should eat 10 grams more of protein, and so on.

Best Protein Sources

- Eggs: whole eggs and egg whites.
- Dairy: milk, Greek yogurt, and cheese.
- Meat: poultry, beef, pork, fish, and seafood. Deli meat is more processed but still a decent option. When cutting, focus on lean meats like chicken breast, turkey, and tuna.
- Legumes: beans, lentils and peas.
- Nuts (and nut butters), seeds, and oats.
- For vegans, soy protein—both in its natural and powder form—might be your best option for getting enough protein. Other sources: beans,

chickpeas, lentils, edamame, peas, bulgur wheat, tofu, barley, oats, rice, quinoa, nuts and nut better, and various seeds like pumpkin and chia.

When to Eat Protein

Space it out throughout the day, so you get protein with every meal. It helps to get at least 20 grams per meal. Your body needs it all day long for protein synthesis, so don't get it all in before noon. Eat three to five times per day, three to five hours apart. Or, have three evenly-spaced meals with protein-rich snacks and shakes in between. A common myth is that you need to consume protein right before or after a workout to build muscle; but as long as you have protein within a few hours of your workout, you're good. For nighttime snacking, casein protein is best, as it is slow-digesting.

Carbs

Carbs are essential for fueling workouts and muscle-building by providing glycogen. According to the Academy of Nutrition and Dietetics, people who strength train at least twice a week need about half of their calories from carbohydrates per day. (Ellis, 2020) Bodybuilders generally consume about this much. (How to Eat Carbs for More Muscle and Less Fat, n.d.) This means that eating low-carb isn't really an option for you, at least while you bulk. The exception is endomorphs who should limit carbs. (Cortes, 2020) Guys of the fat side of skinny-fat might need to limit carbs as well. Mesomorphs can get away with less carbs, but it's optional. Basically, the harder it is for you to gain weight, the more carbs you should eat.

There are two types of carbs, simple and complex. Simple carbs include raw sugar, natural sugar, artificial sweeteners, and corn syrup. They're found in soda, fruit, fruit juice, candy, cereal, baked goods, microwave meals, packaged snacks, and processed grains like white flour. Some of these things, like soda, are useless and should be avoided. However, most simple carbs (especially the naturally occurring ones) do serve a purpose, giving you quick energy right before or during a workout. Eating them right after a workout helps raise your insulin level, to help drive nutrients into the muscles for growth and preventing muscle breakdown. (Hyson, n.d.) A simple piece of fruit will do the job.

Complex carbs are the "good" carbs. They have more nutrients like fiber, vitamins and minerals. They're also slower to digest, spreading your energy more evenly throughout the day. Get them from whole grains, pasta, oats, rice, nuts, beans, vegetables, and fibrous fruit. (Cherney, 2020)

Complex carbs high in starch are often considered the best type of food for post-workout meals. This means potatoes, quinoa, beans, oatmeal, rice, squash, and pasta. If you gain weight easily, eat most of your carbs before, during, and after workouts. Hard-gainers should eat carbs all day, every day.

Finally, you might have heard that white (processed) carbs are bad for you and brown (unprocessed) carbs are good. This might be true for the average (sedentary) person, but plenty of successful athletes and bulkers eat white rice with every meal. Since you'll be doing intense exercise, those simple (processed) carbs will be useful.

Fat

Fat is good for you, *really* good for you. It's essential for providing energy, absorbing vitamins and minerals, building cell membranes, blood clotting, inflammation, and muscle movement. (The Truth About Fats: the Good, the Bad, and the In-betweens, 2019) The American Heart Association recommends healthy adults get about 20 to 35% of total calories from fat. (Zeratsky, 2019)

Like carbs, there's good fats, bad fats, and fats that are iffy. "Good" fat is also known as *unsaturated fat*, both polyunsaturated and monounsaturated. Both are liquid at room temperature. Monounsaturated fats come mostly from vegetables, nuts, seeds, and fish. Good sources of this fat include olive oil, avocados, and most nuts. Polyunsaturated fats are considered "essential" fats, meaning the body needs them but can't naturally produce them. It's found in a variety of fish, seeds, and nuts.

Polyunsaturated fats are also found in many plant-based oils and industrial seed oils, which a growing number of experts agree are terrible for you. They're considered unhealthy for their chemical processing and additives, and their elevated levels of omega-6 fatty acids. (Kresser, 2019) Examples of these oils: vegetable, canola, soybean, corn, cottonseed, peanut, sesame, and sunflower oil.

For guaranteed healthy oils, focus on olive, coconut, and avocado oils. Butter, ghee, lard and tallow are also excellent substitutes.

"Bad" fat is also known as *trans fat*. It should be avoided as well, as a diet laden with trans fat leads to greater risk of heart disease, stroke, and type 2 diabetes. An industrial process called "hydrogenation" turns vegetable oil into a solid to preserve it (aka partially hydrogenated oil). It has essentially zero health benefit, and it's actually banned in the US, but not everywhere in the world. In countries where trans fats are still used, they're prominent in baked goods, shortening, frozen goods, margarine, and fried foods.

Finally, there's *saturated fats*, which experts generally consider "iffy." These are fats that become solid at room temperature, like bacon fat. There's some debate about how healthy they are, and some research has linked it to heart disease. However, other research indicates that it's perfectly fine. (The Truth About Fats: the Good, the Bad, and the In-betweens, 2019) Bacon and eggs have always been a breakfast of champions, and plenty of coaches and trainers continue to recommend saturated fats for their athletes. Common sources of saturated fats include whole milk, fatty red meat cuts, cheese, coconut oil, and many packaged baked goods.

Keep in mind, fat has more calories per gram compared to carbs and protein. That's a good thing when bulking. The more fat you eat, the less total food you'll have to chew. Hard-gainers need to eat lots of it.

Supplements

No supplement is necessary for bulking or cutting, but they can certainly help. I'll mention my four favorites.

Protein powder helps if you can't get enough protein from food. Whether you're building muscle or just maintaining it, you'll need lots of protein, and protein powder will help you get enough. It's safe, and virtually all serious lifters use it (same with protein bars). It also comes in hundreds of different flavors, so it's versatile. I suggest buying small tubs of a few flavors to find what you like, and then you can begin buying the ones you like in bulk. Find it at grocery stores, health food stores, pharmacies, and online.

Creatine also helps aid muscle growth, strength gains, and exercise performance. Interestingly, our bodies can produce creatine naturally from amino acids. When you supplement with it, it provides greater ATP production, which improves your workouts. And, no, despite what you might have heard, creatine is not like steroids. It's one of the most tested supplements in the world and it has an incredible safety record. Still, some people do seem to have a negative reaction to it, such as cramping. Consider adding it to your diet later. If you add it on day one of your new diet with everything else and experience some discomfort, you won't know the cause. Creatine is sold wherever protein powder is sold.

Weight gainers and *meal replacements* are basically liquid meals and they help if you have to eat a lot. They also come in powder form. While protein powder is basically just protein, weight gainer powder is similar to a full meal with a mix of macros and nutrients. Store bought gainer shakes tend to be filled with sugar and other crap, so the healthier option is to make your own.

Vitamin and mineral pills — like one-a-day multivitamins — are safe and effective. The less variety of foods you have in your diet, the more you should consider vitamin pills or powder.

Meal Timing

You're probably used to eating three meals per day, but that might not be enough during a bulk. You'll likely need to at least add in some snacks or shakes between those three meals. A common recommendation is three to five meals a day, spaced out three to five hours between meals. Big bulkers should definitely try this. As long as your calorie intake is spaced pretty evenly throughout the day, then it doesn't really matter at what times you eat. You'll be in a surplus virtually all day. The only exception is, you should eat before workouts if you find yourself lethargic or unfocused working out on an empty stomach.

Chapter 5 Recap

Macros include protein, fat, and carbs. There's lots of wiggle room for how much you get from each category, but you do need all three to build considerable muscle. Choose your macro percentages based on your body type, and consider using "If It Fits Your Macros" if it helps.

Protein is the most important macro for building muscle, and you need at least one gram per pound of bodyweight. Hardgainers might need even more. It's safe, even in much higher quantities. The best protein sources include eggs, dairy, meat, legumes, nuts, seeds, and oats. Vegans have fewer options. Eat protein throughout the day.

Carbs are essential for building muscle. People who gain weight easily should get less carbs (endomorphs and those on the fat side of skinny-fat), while hardgainers need a lot. Mesomorphs have more wiggle room. Simple carbs are useful but should be used sparingly, mostly during and near workouts, while complex carbs are generally healthier.

Fat is an essential macro and you should get around 20-35% of total calories from it. Fat has more calories per gram compared to other macros. Focus on eating the good fats (while avoiding unhealthy oils), avoid the bad fats, and be careful with saturated fats. Supplements aren't essential but I recommend four: protein powder, creatine, weight gainer, and vitamin/mineral pills. Try to eat four to five meals per day.

CHAPTER 6: MEAL PLANNING

If you're going to cook your meals instead of having take-out and delivery, I strongly recommend planning out your meals ahead of time. Make a grocery list with everything you'll need for the week, and have all the necessary kitchen utensils and ingredients at hand.

Your off days—the days you don't work out—are the best time to take care of this stuff. You don't want to wake up one morning and realize you have to make a bunch of decisions about food on top of having to go grind in the gym.

Some bulkers prefer to stick to only a few recipes. Some even eat the same exact meals every day, which makes shopping and buying in bulk much easier. You might prefer more variety, though.

I'll list a few meal plan ideas and shake recipes below. However, I won't be providing a comprehensive meal plan. Ultimately, it's better that you find recipes you like that fit within the foods and macros that you know are best for you. That way, you'll learn what you like, how to choose and combine ingredients, and how to form a better habit of planning your own meals.

The internet is full of free recipes for every type of diet. Search based on macro priority—high protein, low carb, etc.—or simply search for "healthy calorie dense meals." The subreddit r/gainitmeals is a goldmine for healthy, high-calorie recipes.

See this list at allrecipes.com (allrecipes.com/recipes/84/healthy-recipes/) to find healthy meal ideas. This page from clevelandclinic.org (https://cle.clinic/34ee41F) has great ideas for healthy, high-calorie snacks.

Meal Prep

This usually means setting aside one day per week to make several meals, and keep them in Tupperware for on-the-go eating. You can cook several pounds of meat, rice, vegetables, and other bulk goods. Simply assemble individual meals into containers, put them in the refrigerator, and warm up when it's time to eat.

You can prep snacks too. Fill Ziplock bags with healthy snacks to-go: baby carrots, mixed nuts, etc. Or pack whole sandwiches: lunch meat and cheese PB&J, etc.

There are some basic kitchen utensils you'll want to own:

- Kitchen knife
- Cutting board
- Pot and pan
- Spatula
- Stirring spoon
- Baking pan
- Measuring cups
- Can opener
- Tongs
- Colander
- Peeler

Essential ingredients you'll probably want to have on hand:

- Oil, vinegar, and condiments: soy sauce, hot sauce, mustard, mayo, etc.
- Seasonings: salt, pepper, dried herbs, cinnamon, vanilla, etc.
- Baking products: baking powder, baking soda, flour, sugar, honey, etc.
- Canned goods: beans, peanut butter, jelly, tomatoes, tuna, salsa, etc.
- Grains and legumes: rice, oats, pasta, etc.
- Refrigerator goods: butter, cheese, eggs, yogurt, etc.
- Freeezer goods: fruits and vegetables.
- Produce: onion, garlic, potatoes, nuts and seeds, and dried fruit.

You'll want to learn various cooking techniques too. Heating everything in the microwave will get old really fast. Some basic techniques you can explore:

- Making stew (or almost anything else) in a crock pot
- Roasting chicken and baking fish in the oven
- Making rice in a pot or rice cooker
- Scrambling or frying eggs in a pan
- Stir-frying rice and protein bowls
- Slicing and roasting vegetables

- Grilling panini sandwiches
- Searing steak
- Boiling pasta

You can also learn to use an outdoor grill or smoker and make virtually every meal with it. Same goes for cast-iron pans.

Learning to cook is like learning anything else; you get the basics down, and then you can experiment with what you like. It's like learning to play guitar: you learn a few chords, practice a little each day, and then one day something just clicks and you're suddenly *getting it*.

Use YouTube and search for what you need: "Beginners guide to cooking," "How to Use a Cast Iron," "Crockpot Basics," or "Grilling 101." Most top search results will have millions of views and are filled with useful nuggets of cooking wisdom that I couldn't say better myself.

Fast Food

As a general rule, fast-food isn't the healthiest or most "optimal" option, but that's not how life works. Some days, your only choice will be to stop in at a local fast-food place and grab something quick. However, that doesn't mean you can't order something relatively healthy. Below are a few healthy (to healthy-ish) options from popular fast-food joints:

- Burrito bowls: found at most Mexican food joints like Taco Bell and Chipotle, filled with protein and vegetables (same with regular burritos).
- Breakfast wraps/sandwiches: Starbucks, Dunkin', Subway, and McDonalds have options with eggs, vegetables, and whole-grains. Other places (like Chick-fil-A) have a grilled chicken option.
- Burgers: Plenty of protein and vegetables, skip the sauces, and even nix the buns for less carbs. In n Out has a "protein style" burger wrapped in lettuce, which is a lot easier than using a fork and knife.
- Grilled chicken wraps and burgers: Find these at Sonic, Chick-fil-A, McDonalds, and several other places.
- Sandwiches: Subway is king. You can add double meat, pack on the vegetables, and opt for the healthier sauces.

- Salads: These are almost ubiquitous these days; Wendy's, Subway, Panera, Chick-fil-A, Arby's, Del Taco, and more.
- Asian bowls: Panda Express and others have plenty of high-protein, vegetable-rich, and clean-carb options.
- Pizza: a mix of high-protein sources and fresh vegetables.
- Ordering take out: depending on the restaurant, you have a ton of healthy options. There's steak, fajitas, grilled chicken, chili, soup, sushi, poke bowls, and so much more. Healthy sides include salad (lite or no dressing), vegetables, loaded potatoes, fruit bowls, and whatever else contains whole ingredients and fits your macros.

Dorm Room Bulk

If you live in a dorm or a similar situation where you don't have a full kitchen, you'll have to improvise. Obviously, if your school has a cafeteria, take advantage of it. Not everyone will have that option, though.

Below are some meals you can make in the dorm with just a mini-fridge and microwave (or hot plate).

Breakfast:

Muesli with Greek yogurt, oats, raisins, hazelnuts, and apple
Overnight oatmeal with milk, blueberries, and honey
Microwave oatmeal with cinnamon and butter
Microwave scrambled eggs with hot sauce
Low-sugar, high-protein cereal with milk
No-bake muffins with oats and berries

Lunch:

Greens salad with avocado and cherry tomatoes
Ham sandwich + Greek yogurt + apple
Sardines, crackers, and hot sauce
Hummus and veggie wrap

Meal replacement shake
PB&J + banana

Dinner:

Microwave instant rice with black beans, avocado, and cheese
Microwave frozen vegetable bag with microwave baked potato
Rotisserie chicken from grocery store (it's warm and cheap)
Canned tuna with mayo, relish, and whole wheat crackers
Canned vegetables with canned chicken and Sriracha
Spinach and canned chicken salad

Snacks:

Whole wheat crackers and cream cheese
Cottage cheese and canned peaches
Greek yogurt, granola, and walnuts
Peanut butter and apple or celery
Canned fruit salad and yogurt
Frozen yogurt with berries
Hummus and carrots
Protein shake or bar
Fresh or dried fruit
Mixed nuts
Beef jerky

Blender Bulk

Shakes are incredibly convenient and portable. Hard-gainers will probably
need at least one per day. The best ones are dense in calories, rich in protein, and
low in sugar. The most basic protein shakes require only protein powder and a
shaker cup sold at most grocery stores. Mass gainer shakes require a blender. See
this   infographic   from   the   subreddit   r/gainitmeals

(https://i.redd.it/bplc6sxqsh541.png) for tons of shake recipes including vegan and gluten-free options.

Below are a few more shake ideas from the subreddit "Gain It" (reddit.com/r/gainit):

1,000 Cal Milk & Honey:

Ingredients: 1 scoop protein, 1/2 cup oats, 1/2 cup whole milk, 1/2 cup half & half, 1/8 cup peanut butter, 1 tablespoon Honey, 1 tablespoon Nutella, 1 banana. Total calories: roughly 1,000.

The 1K Cal Breakfast:

2 cups of whole milk, 2 packets strawberries and creme instant oatmeal, 2 scoops vanilla protein powder, half a cup full fat Greek yogurt, 12 tablespoons (200 ml) egg whites, 2 tablespoon olive oil. Total calories: 1,313 (Protein: 107g, Carbs: 93g, Fat: 59g).

The 1,700 Calorie Cup:

2 cups whole milk (300 kcal), 1 1/2 cups ground dry oats (450 kcal), 2 scoops whey protein (260 kcal), 1 cup full fat Greek yogurt (220 kcal), 30 ground almonds (300 kcal), 1 tablespoon coconut oil (120 kcal), 1 large banana (70 kcal). Total calories: 1,720.

Super Green:

Water, 2 scoops grass-fed whey, 1 cup walnuts, 1 1/2 cups spinach, 1 banana, 1/4 avocado, 1/2 apple, 1 tablespoon coconut oil. Total calories: 986 (Protein: 35g, Sugar: 31g).

2 Meals in One Cup:

1 cup oats, 6 ounces Honey, half a cup Greek yogurt, 1 tablespoon olive oil, 2 tablespoons peanut butter, 5g creatine, 2 scoops banana weight gainer powder, 2 cups whole milk, 1 cup raw almonds. Grind almonds with oats into a powder before combining with the rest. Total calories: 2,938.

Paleo Shake:

1/2 cup mixed nuts (grind into powder first), 2 scoops pure coconut oil, 1 banana or scoop of berries, 1 scoop protein powder, 1 cup coconut milk, 1 cup almond milk, 1/2 cup water. Total calories: 975 (Fat: 69g, Protein: 45g, Carbs: 51g).

Orange Creamsicle:

1 cup whole milk, 1/2 cup heavy cream, 3 cups orange juice, 6 raw eggs, 1 teaspoon vanilla. Total calories: 1,180.

The 30-Second Shake:

3 cups water or milk, 2 scoops whey protein powder, and ice. Add a diet root beer or orange soda for a kick.

Bulking on A Budget

Despite what you may have heard, *eating healthy is not expensive* and you don't have to shop at high-end specialty stores. Your regular local grocery store or a discount membership warehouse will do. Here are some tips to keep in mind:

1. Buy in bulk, especially when it comes to quality meats, vegetables, fruits, grains, cooking oils, spices, and sauces. Some things you'll only have to buy once every few months, others once a week.
2. Buy the generic store brands to save even more. Often the generic product is the exact same actual food as the name brand, especially when it comes to highly marked-up milk.

3. Take advantage of sales to stock up.

Below is a grocery list that proves just how cheap eating healthy can be.

Bulking On $50 Per Week

(Numbers based on 2019 Walmart prices, generic products when available, and bought in bulk when available)

4 lbs. boneless, skinless chicken breast (1,760 cal, 320g protein): $7.98
2 lbs. ground beef (1,920 cal, 168g protein): $7.24
1 lb. uncooked whole grain rice (1,710 cal, 38g protein): $1.69
3 dozen eggs (2,520 cal, 216g protein): $4.50
1 gallon whole milk (2,400 cal, 128g protein): $3.28
4 lbs. (approx. 14) bananas (1,470 cal, 18g protein): $2.16
2 cans black beans (630 cal, 42g protein): $1.44
20 oz. natural peanut butter (3,230 cal, 119g protein): $2.82
21 oz. whole grain oatmeal (2,250 cal, 75g protein): $1.24
4 lbs. frozen mixed vegetables (1,100 cal, 44g protein): $4.44
2 cans tuna (360 cal, 80g protein): $2.00
1 lb. whey protein powder, (1,680 cal, 336g protein): $10.53

- Total Calories: 21,030 (3,004 per day)
- Total Protein: 1,584g (226g per day)
- *Total Cost: $49.32*

$75 Per Week

Now let's add some more items to the above list:

1 loaf (24 oz) whole grain bread (1,800 cal, 75g protein): $1.98
1 jar (4.25 oz) sugar free jelly (70 cal, 0g protein): $0.94
1 can (13 oz) mixed nuts (2,210 cal, 78g protein): $4.20
1 bag (2.3 oz) dried fruit variety pack (250 cal, 2g protein): $4.48

1 lb. bacon (800 cal, 56g protein): $4.32
1 bottle (8 oz) extra virgin olive oil (1,920 cal, 0g protein): $2.06
5 Hass avocados (1,200 cal, 15g protein): $2.90
1 tub (32 oz) nonfat vanilla Greek yogurt (450 cal, 70g protein): $3.73

Adds: 8,700 cal, 296g protein, $24.61.

Both Lists Combined:

- Total Calories: 29,730 (4,247 per day)
- Total Protein: 1,880g (269g per day)
- *Total Cost: $73.93*

Chapter 6 Recap

Plan your meals ahead of time, and have all necessary ingredients and kitchen equipment on hand before you bulk. Take care of meal planning on off days. You might consider setting aside one day per week to prepare all of your meals for the upcoming week.

You can eat the same stuff every day or have more variety. It will help you tremendously to learn over time which recipes you like, how to prepare them, and how to form healthy eating habits. Use the internet for recipes, snack ideas, and cooking instructions.

You can bulk even if you don't have access to a full kitchen and I provide lots of examples of meals and shakes you can prepare even in a dorm room. Bulking can also be done very cheaply, even for $75 per week.

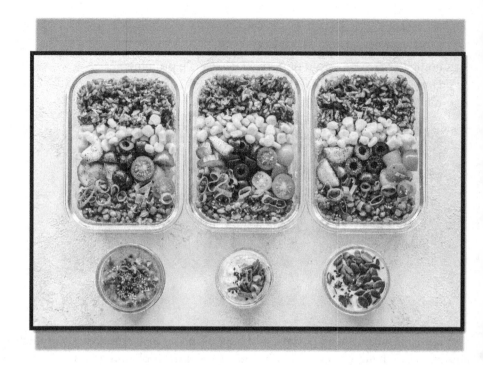

PART 2: BULKING AND CUTTING

CHAPTER 7: THE SMALL AND NORMAL BULKS

Like I mentioned in a previous chapter, unless you're obese, then the only way you can gain muscle mass (at a reasonable pace) is to gain weight, and the only way to gain weight is to eat more calories than you're burning. In strength training this is known as "bulking." How many calories you should bulk with depends on a few key factors: your age, body type, current body composition, and how close you already are to your genetic potential for muscle gains. Skinny hardgainers will likely require the "big bulk," which I'll discuss in the next chapter. Most guys will be best off with a small or normal bulk, so let's look at them in detail.

The Small Bulk

This means eating a daily surplus of *200 to 300 calories*. So if your maintenance calories (including the small increase from your new workouts) are 2,400, then you would eat 2,600 to 2,700 kcal per day. That's an addition of around 10% of your maintenance calories. The upside to this choice is that you'll gain less fat and you don't have to eat a ton of food. The downside is you'll likely gain muscle slower and the bulk will last longer, from months to a year or more. A small bulk typically means a gain of 1% of your body weight per month. It's best for:

1. Guys who gain weight easily but aren't obese. Usually endomorphs and those on the fat side of skinny-fat. Still, some shouldn't bulk at all.
2. Most guys 35 and older.
3. Advanced trainees (meaning, you've been lifting for several years).
4. Intermediate trainees who are happy with how they look but would like to keep making slow and steady gains (and minimal fat gain).

Most men will have some level of success with a small bulk, but it's more appropriate for some than others. The small bulk is usually the best choice for middle-aged guys, because your body won't respond as well to a bigger bulk. Some men past 35 can get away with eating much more than this, but as a general rule, it's smart to play it safe. If you bulk more than this, you might gain muscle faster, but you'll also likely gain more fat than others. It's also best for more advanced weightlifters, especially those who don't want to lose their six-pack (very advanced lifters might need an even smaller surplus of 100 kcal or less).

A 2010 study from the Norwegian School of Sports Medicine monitored a group of strength-trained athletes for an 8- to 12-week period. One group ate a specific amount (roughly 500 kcal surplus) while the other group ate whatever they wanted (they ate less). They all gained roughly the same amount of lean mass, but the group that ate more gained way more bodyweight and fat. Therefore, being that they were all well-trained athletes (already near their muscular potential), there was no added benefit to eating more than necessary. The researchers speculated that a 200-300 kcal surplus is better for elite athletes than a 500 kcal surplus when the additional weight gain is of no benefit. (Garthe, 2010)

If you are an endomorph who has recently lost weight (i.e. you're no longer obese but you can still easily gain weight) and you want to bulk up, you might benefit from a very small bulk. Although, I'd recommend eating maintenance calories and lifting weights until you achieve a better body composition (especially if you are already over 15% BF). Then you can bulk. The same goes for guys that are skinny-fat and still have bodyfat over 15%. A recomp might last only a couple of months, and once you're at a better bodyfat level, you should be in a much better position to bulk up for faster gains.

With the small bulk, you can expect a gain of half a pound of bodyweight per week at most, although it might be at only half that rate. The small bulk will also have a muscle to fat gain ratio of 1:1 or better. That is, you might gain much more muscle than bodyfat, but you'll gain it much slower than other bulkers. This type of bulk is often called a "lean bulk," because you'll typically gain minimal fat compared to muscle.

If you aren't gaining weight, if your lifts aren't improving, or if the progress slows down, add an extra 100 kcal per week until you're gaining weight and strength steadily. If you feel your fat gain is too much, reduce to maintenance calories and see if you can build a little muscle.

How long this small bulk will last will depend on your goals and how well you can add muscle. If you want to get truly jacked, it could take several months to a few years. Gaining weight at a rate of half a pound per week (at best) would mean gaining around 26 pounds in a year (with half or more of those gains being muscle). If you can't wait that long (and you're willing to gain more fat in the short-term), consider if this next type of bulk might be appropriate for you. In the next section, I'll also discuss the rate at which you can expect to build muscle with more detail.

A final note about the small bulk: the smaller the surplus you shoot for, the more precision it takes with your diet. As an example, let's say you decide to bulk with a 100-cal surplus because you think it's the absolute minimum surplus you need to build some muscle. You want to avoid fat gain as much as possible, so you're willing to gain muscle very slowly.

Eating exactly 100 kcal over maintenance is a tight-rope walk, and it's very easy to shoot over or under that. It will take extreme discipline to hit that exact amount every day, and if you ever go under, you won't gain (in this example). Go over, and you'll gain more fat than you wanted. This is one reason (among many) why some folks will prefer the next bulk, which allows a little more error.

The Normal Bulk

This means eating a surplus of about *400 to 600 calories*. This is an increase of around 20% of your maintenance calories. Compared to a small bulk, you'll eat a little more and add a little more muscle and fat. It's worth it if you'd rather gain muscle faster (perhaps twice as fast) and have a shorter bulk.

The small and normal bulks represent the most common recommendation for gaining size. That is, around 10 to 20% of maintenance calories. Beginners will usually do better around 20%, while more advanced lifters will do better closer to 10%.

A 2019 study headed by sports nutritionist Juma Iraki found that novice/intermediate bodybuilders will gain around 0.25-0.5% of bodyweight per week (1-2% of bodyweight per month) on a diet in the 10-20% range. (Iraki et al., 2019) So if your maintenance calories are 2,500 per day, then you'd eat 2,750 to 3,000 per day, respectively. Eating in the 20% range (a normal bulk), a 180-pound man would gain roughly 0.5-1lb per week (2-4lbs per month).

Consider that it takes roughly 3,500 extra calories to gain one pound of bodyweight. (Counting Calories: Get Back to Weight-Loss Basics, 2020) Therefore, if you eat 500 extra calories per day, then (theoretically) you should gain about one pound per week. Really though, it depends on your macros. Dietary fat stores as bodyfat more easily than do protein or carbs. Also, building and storing muscle via protein synthesis requires more energy than simply storing fat. (Satrazemis, 2019)

Your muscle-gain to fat-gain will likely be around 1:1, meaning you'll gain about one pound of muscle for every one pound of new fat. Although, some estimates put it at a much more favorable rate with less fat gain. A 2019 study out the University of Northern Parana found that a group of bodybuilders who ate 4,500 kcal per day (by no means a small bulk) gained at a rate of 4:1. Meaning, they gained only one pound of bodyfat for every four pounds of muscle gained. (Ribeiro et al., 2019)

Renowned strength training coach Mark Rippetoe believes it's more like 60% muscle gain and 40% fat gain for beginners. That's an excellent ratio. Total weight gain will likely be around 2% of your body weight per month. So if you weigh 175lbs, you'd gain roughly 3.5lbs your first month, or around a pound per week. You'd be about 10lbs heavier in three months.

The normal bulk is best for:

1. Any beginner or intermediate with normal body weight and BF% who's willing to gain more fat in exchange for quicker muscle gains than a small bulk allows.
2. Young guys on the skinny side of skinny-fat. If over 35, try the small bulk first.

If you've ever scoured bulking sites and instructional videos, you know that eating 500 extra calories is a very common tip for bulkers. That's because it's a nice middle ground between eating just enough to gain relatively fast without gaining too much fat. Still, it's not best for everyone. Advanced trainees shouldn't use it as they are so close to their genetic potential and can't gain muscle fast enough to justify a normal bulk. If you're a beginner or intermediate who would benefit from a small bulk, you will almost certainly gain more muscle (and fat) on a normal bulk.

Very skinny guys (hardgainers) will likely need more calories than a normal bulk calls for, while guys under 35 on the skinny side of skinny-fat (meaning you're skinny but have a little bit of belly fat) should try the normal bulk first and only exceed it if necessary.

How long does the normal bulk last? Again, it depends. You might find after only a few months to a year that you're able to reduce calories and continue bulking and gaining muscle. Intermediates might even be happy with their gains after a year or so, and at that point they can transition from a bulk to a recomp or cut. Or, you might get to that point and decide you want to keep going for more gains. Regardless, after those first few months, you'll likely require less calories to recover from training. In other words, you'll keep bulking but with a smaller surplus. This will be near the point where you graduate from beginner to intermediate, too, and that's when you have a lot of training options going forward.

Add the Surplus Slowly

Let's say you've decided a 500 kcal surplus is right for you. You shouldn't add them all to your diet on day one. It's better to add a little at a time, perhaps 100 to 200 per week, for a few reasons: you'll give you body time to slowly adjust to the full surplus, and more importantly, you might not even need the full 500 kcal surplus. Let's say you add 150 kcal daily for the first week and your lifts are improving. The weight isn't very heavy yet, but you're feeling fatigued and you missed a rep or two. The second week you add another 150 kcal. Now you're recovering even better, your lifts are progressing like they should, and you're starting to gain weight quicker.

It's possible at this point, you're eating enough, and you don't need to add to your 300 kcal surplus. If instead, you added all 500 kcal on day one, you'll start gaining weight quickly and your strength will improve workout-to-workout. But we know all you needed was 300 extra calories, so you're going to be gaining more weight and bodyfat than necessary. A big downside to this is that after a few months, the fat gain might be so much that you have no choice but to lose some fat on a cut or recomp. The weeks it takes you to lose the fat are weeks you'll be missing out on some insane gains.

How Fast and How Much You Can Gain

Fitness author Lye McDonald compared various models for muscular gain potential and came up with these estimates: beginner males (using a moderate bulk) can expect to gain 1.5 to 2 pounds of muscle per month for the first year. Keep in mind, for every pound of muscle gain, you'll likely gain up to a pound of fat as well. Therefore, in your first year of consistent bulking and strength training, you'd gain 20 to 25 pounds of muscle (up to 40 to 50 pounds of total bodyweight). Your second year more like 10 to 12 pounds of muscle, your third year 5 to 6 pounds of muscle, and 2 to 3 pounds of muscle for all years after that. (McDonald, 2009)

Of course, these are best-case-scenario numbers. The further you are from your prime (late teens to early twenties), the less you can gain. A forty-year-old man probably won't gain 25 pounds of muscle in a year. Some younger men might have a better muscle-to-fat-gain ratio than 1:1. Underweight men especially might gain even more muscle than these numbers suggest. Of course, if you're underweight, then you're probably a skinny hardgainer, and you'll likely require even more calories to build muscle (i.e. the big bulk.).

The average man can expect to gain 40 to 50 pounds of muscle in his life, and he can often reach close to this upper limit within 4 or 5 years of consistent training and bulking. (Matthews, Here's How Much Muscle You Can Really Gain Naturally) Of course, this assumes you're "natty" and not using steroids. If you've heard stories of celebrities gaining 40 pounds of muscle in a year for a new superhero role, steroids are probably involved.

If you want to get a decent idea of how much muscle you'll be able to gain over your lifetime, find a "natural muscular potential calculator" online. It will ask for your height, bodyfat, and the size of your wrists and ankles. The estimate of 40 to 50 pounds of muscle gains over a lifetime is for the average man, not all men. Underweight males usually stand to gain even more.

The First Few Weeks of Bulking

If you're a beginner to strength training, you'll get stronger very fast during the first few weeks to months. This is due to your nervous system improving at handling heavy weights as you also gain muscle. Combined, these are referred to as "newbie gains," which I'll explain in more detail later.

Another interesting thing that might happen early on in your training is your muscles might get stronger but not bigger. According to sports scientist and powerlifter Greg Nuckols, you likely won't gain muscular size during your first two to three weeks of training. During this period, the best your muscles can do is repair themselves. He says you should expect it to take around a month of consistent training before you see a visual difference in muscle gains and two to three months before seeing truly noticeable changes. (Nuckols, 2017)

Basically, during your first two or three weeks of training, your muscles will get denser and stronger, guaranteed. But it might take up to four weeks for them to grow in size. By month two or three, they'll be obviously bigger.

Track Your Progress

You'll need to keep track of your weight gain from day one. Once you are consuming your target surplus, you can start making any needed adjustments to food intake.

If you're doing a small bulk, aim to gain around 0.25 to 0.5 pounds per week. If you're doing a normal bulk, aim for 0.5 to 1 pound of weight gain per week. As long as you're hitting those numbers, and your strength training is on track, then you're on the right path.

If you aren't gaining weight after the first week, add 100 kcal and track your progress for another week. Keep adding calories once a week until you start gaining weight. If, on the other hand, you're gaining weight too quickly, consider dropping your calories by 100. Try it for a week, reassess, and keep reducing calories until you're comfortable with your rate of weight gain.

Just keep tweaking your calories based on what you see on the scale, in the mirror, and in the gym. It's more of an art than a science. Remember that the whole point of gaining weight is to put muscle on your body, and the best way to know if you're building muscle is if your lifts are improving workout-to-workout. If you're a beginner, the first few weeks to months will include "newb gains," meaning your nervous system is getting stronger. If you stop gaining strength after the newb gains dwindle, then you're not building muscle. If this happens, you need more calories or changes to your training.

Finally, there's no need to measure your weight every day. Your weight will fluctuate daily, so a little gain or loss day-to-day won't tell you much. It's better to measure your weight gain once a week, preferably first thing in the morning after peeing.

Chapter 7 Recap

Most bulkers will require one of these two moderate bulks. With the "small bulk," you'll eat a daily surplus of 200 to 300 kcal, and you can expect to gain 0.25 to 0.5 pounds per week. It's best for anyone with a high bodyfat percentage or who gains weight easily, advanced trainees, and most men over 35. Adjust your calories based on how your lifts are improving and how you look in the mirror. The bulk will likely last several months and can go longer depending on your goals.

With the "normal bulk," you'll eat a daily surplus 400 to 600 kcal. You should gain muscle and fat at around a 1:1 ratio (or better), and you'll gain half to one pound of bodyweight per week. It's best for people with normal body weight and bodyfat percentage who want quicker gains than a small bulk allows, guys on the skinny-fat side of skinny, and most beginner and intermediate trainees. This bulk should last at least a few months, but you might extend it depending on your goals.

Best case scenario is you'll gain 25 pounds of muscle your first year. Older guys won't gain this much, and hardgainers will require more calories to get these gains. Always track your weight gain by measuring weight once per week. Add or subtract 100 kcal per week as needed.

CHAPTER 8: HOW HARDGAINERS CAN ADD MASS FAST: THE BIG BULK

This bulk is for young, naturally-skinny, hard-gainer beginners only. **No one else.**

The purpose of this bulk is to help kickstart a growth spurt for those who have a very hard time gaining weight and have the potential to add a ton of weight and muscle. I'm talking about you guys who can eat everything in sight and still look like you weigh ninety pounds soaking wet.

It requires a daily surplus of anywhere from *700 to 1,000 calories or even more*. To be clear, you have to be very careful with this type of bulk. Weight gain can happen rapidly, especially fat gain. You can expect to gain weight at a rate of about one to two pounds per week (or higher). The more underweight you are, the faster you'll gain. Eventually, your body will fill out, you'll no longer be underweight, and you can reduce calories to more of a normal bulk to keep gaining.

Just like the small and normal bulks, you should be shooting for a fat-gain to muscle-gain ratio of 1:1 or better. Being that you're starting off so skinny, there's a good chance that you'll gain much less fat than muscle, and your ratio will be way better than 1:1. You might gain two or three times as much muscle than fat for your first few months. However, as you fill out and stop being underweight (usually around the two month mark) your gain ratio will become closer to 1:1.

Why Hardgainers Should Gain Fast

Taller and leaner folks (who start underweight) can easily gain ten pounds of bodyweight per month for the first few months. At that rate, assuming you're training and recovering correctly, then you're likely gaining more muscle than fat. However, even gaining at a 1:1 ratio, that's five pounds of muscle in a month. Pretty incredible! And it's very doable for a hardgainer (I'll explain why in a minute). Even if it's five pounds of fat gain, it's a good thing to add lots of weight quickly when you start off underweight. In fact, being at a very low weight and bodyfat percentage might prevent you from building any muscle.

According to exercise physiologist Mike Nelson, low bodyfat levels lead to low glycogen levels, which are vital to muscle repair and recovery. (Fetters, 15 Negative Effects of Having a Low Body-fat Percentage) The extra fat will also help aid your new training, protect your joints for the big lifts, and you'll certainly look better. Besides, in your case, you can gain plenty more bodyfat before you even approach being legitimately obese. You won't get a big Santa belly after only a couple of months.

Other reasons adding a ton of calories can help: you remain in a calorie surplus throughout the day, which helps with protein synthesis and recovery; and the extra weight gain and the resulting higher levels of testosterone will also help build muscle. The fact is, when you're a total beginner (aka a rank novice) and you start off very underweight, it is necessary to add lots of weight (perhaps 20lbs in two months) as your lower body lifts improve by 100 to 150lbs.

Remember, this is the whole point of gaining weight! Without the added weight, you can miss reps and fail to progress in the gym. Since these are the fastest gains a man will ever experience, it seems better to not worry about the fat gain for the time being. It's worth it. These first two or three months of big bulking will likely put you over the "ideal" 15% bodyfat mark (perhaps closer to 20%), but that's not the end of the world. You're not obese, and you can lose the extra fat later. One thing's for sure, this is no time to start thinking about doing a cut or recomp, which will only see you miss out on once-in-a-lifetime gains.

There's no question that eating a high-calorie diet is the best way to get more gains. As sports scientist Dr. Mike Israetel explains it, "The single most important change you can make to your diet to gain more muscle is to eat more food. It's that simple. All else being equal, eating more is the most powerful tool for muscle gain, as long as you're training hard."

Luckily, this huge calorie surplus won't be required for long, depending on how much muscle you stand to gain and how underweight you are to begin with. It will likely take around two months of consistently overeating with this huge surplus for your body to fill out. After that, you'll be able to eat gradually less while still recovering from workouts and building muscle (at a slower rate). This will also ensure that you don't start gaining way more fat than muscle. You might get all the way down to a small 200 to 300 calorie surplus after several months, while continuing to pack on muscle.

Again, you shouldn't add all of those extra calories at once. You can add an extra 200+ weekly until you hit your desired bulk. You can begin strength training while you ramp up the calories. If you do it this way, then the closer you get to eating your target surplus, the faster you'll gain weight. So if you want to gain 2+ pounds per week, don't expect it to happen until you're eating the full big bulk surplus. Plus, you might find that you're eating enough before hitting the full surplus of 1,000 kcal or whatever your target was.

How Fast Should I Gain Weight?

How fast you should gain weight depends on how fast you can gain muscle, which depends on your genetics, age, and training history. The younger and less trained you are, and the further you are from your genetic potential, the quicker you can gain. First, let's talk about the average adult male (not specifically hardgainers).

According to Nate Miyaki, C.S.S.N., a nutrition coach to physique competitors, a male beginner in his teens up through his thirties can expect to put on two to four pounds of lean muscle per month, for the first two or three months of his training (and a slower gain rate for the rest of the first year). An intermediate trainee (several months' to a few years' experience) might see 1 to 1.5 pounds per month. An advanced lifter, on the other hand, should be happy with just a few pounds per year. (How to Build Muscle: The Best Muscle-building Diet, n.d.)

These numbers are supported by the 2010 Norwegian School of Sports Medicine study, where researchers believed a maximal increase in lean body mass of .55-1.1lbs per week may be realistic. This would come out to 2.2-4.4lbs of lean mass gains per month. The researchers suggested a daily surplus of 500-1,000 kcal might be optimal to achieve these gains. However, they noted that athletes with a long history of strength training would likely have less ability to add so much lean mass. (Garthe, 2010)

In the best-case scenario, the *average* young beginner would gain roughly 12 pounds of muscle— potentially 24 pounds total body weight if he gains muscle and fat at 1:1—in the first three months. But this is unlikely if you don't meet the right criteria: young, true beginner, etc. Keep in mind, this is only for the first few months of training when you'll experience the faster rate of muscle gains.

Okay, But How Fast Will a Hardgainer Gain?

Now, here's the twist. The studies mentioned above applied to young beginners in general, but not specifically to skinny hardgainers. Plenty of studies have demonstrated that the *average* young beginner can realistically gain up to two pounds of muscle per month for the first year (potentially twice that rate during the first few months). Those are incredible "newbie gains." However, we know from the experience of coaches and trainers (and from the testimonials of men who have done it) that young hardgainers can often gain lean mass *even faster*. In fact, a 2005 study out of Indiana University (IUPUI) demonstrated that some guys can gain muscle up to three times as fast as the average. (Hubal, 2005)

This is due to the fact that most adult males have a decent amount of muscle mass naturally. This means they are already closer to their genetic potential than a young hardgainer who has much less muscle on his body. Therefore, when your average Joe begins training, he doesn't stand to gain as much muscle mass as the skinny guy who is starting closer to zero.

This is the reason why some skinny hardgainers can eat twice the calories of a normal bulk and not get especially fat. Because he can potentially get twice the gains! You see, you're not eating 1,000+ kcal just so that you can gain twice the fat as other guys, you're actually building muscle faster. At least, some hardgainers will, but results will vary wildly.

When to Eat More for Better Gains

Let's use a hypothetical: Andrew is 25 years old, 6'0, and weighs 160lbs (super skinny). He's a total newb to strength training, he struggles to gain weight, and his daily maintenance calories are 2,500. He decides to begin his bulk at 3,300 kcal (800 surplus), and he starts a lifting program, lifting three times per week. For his first month of bulking and training, let's say he gains six pounds of body weight—most being muscle, while some is surely fat—and he can see that his body is filling out nicely. His lifts are progressing in the gym, but he did miss a few reps during his workouts recently.

It has Andrew wondering if he might not be eating enough, so he decides to add more calories to get even faster gains. He ramps it up to 3,500 kcal, and the second month he gains another eight pounds of bodyweight. He also didn't fail on any lifts, he's recovering nicely from every workout, and he's not looking particularly fluffy in the mirror. Now the question is, was the increase in calories from 3,300 to 3,500 necessary? Did he get even get faster muscle gains or did he just accelerate the fat gains?

In this situation, you have to decide if you felt a real surge in strength and whether your lifts have had a marked improvement since upping the calories in the second month. Tracking your gym progress will help with this. You should also have a decent idea of whether you've gained fat even faster as a result. This you'll have to determine by simply looking in the mirror and being honest with the changes you've seen in your appearance. Taking occasional progress pictures will help with this. (This is assuming you don't have regular access to the precise but expensive bodyfat machines in sports clinics and doctor offices.).

Or maybe you don't care as much about the extra fat gain. If you're happy to gain more fat in exchange for faster muscle gains, then you should be satisfied knowing that the extra calories might have improved your lifts and gave you better muscle gains. They also might not have helped, but you feel better safe than sorry. You know that you definitely didn't leave any gains on the table by not eating enough.

This logic might seem reckless to some, but when you start off underweight like Andrew did, you'll probably look awesome with that extra 14 pounds after just two months. You're not obese, or even close to it; at worst (as a result of upping the calories in month two) you gained an extra pound or two of fat that you can just burn off in a week if you eventually do a cut. By eating at the higher end of the big bulk range, then you know your diet isn't the issue when something eventually goes wrong with your training program and you starting missing reps. You'll know that it's something else, such as not resting enough between sets or using bad form.

Another benefit to choosing to eat more is, when you eventually eat less than you meant to (say you're shooting for a 1,000-kcal surplus but you accidentally eat only 800 one day), that won't prevent you from building muscle. You might build it at a slightly slower pace, but you're still gaining. It's when your surplus is small that missing a couple hundred calories can prevent any and all gains. For example, if a 500-calorie surplus is optimal for your gains, and one day you eat only 200 extra calories, that's a big enough drop-off that you might get zero gains.

Add Calories Carefully

Of course, this logic shouldn't lead you to just keep adding more and more calories. If you do keep ramping up your calories, you'll eventually hit a point of diminishing returns, and you'll start gaining too much fat. Remember, you can only build muscle so fast. You have to find that "sweet spot" between too few calories and too many.

If you're gaining more than two pounds of body weight per week, you should assess your body and consider reducing calories. Still, it's possible you really are gaining more muscle than fat at that pace. If you're gaining less than two pounds per week but the fat gain seems out of control, or you don't notice an improvement in training, you should also reduce calories.

If you're getting stronger—able to lift heavier things as your workout program requires—and gaining some weight week-to-week, you're eating enough. Sure, you might be leaving some gains on the table by not eating even more, but as long as you're happy with your gains, then you're eating enough. If you aren't getting stronger or gaining weight, increase calories. If you're gaining weight but not getting stronger, you're not building muscle, and it's an issue of not eating the right stuff or not training correctly.

How to Be Sure You're Right for the Big Bulk

Again, I recommend the big bulk only for those who meet all of the following criteria: taller men under age 35, who are underweight with naturally low bodyfat (i.e. ectomorphs), who have a hard time gaining weight, and who are beginners to training. These are the hardest of hard-gainers. In this case, the big bulk is likely the only type of bulk that will work for you.

If you are all of the above, except that you're closer to skinny-fat than skinny, be extra careful. Consider beginning with a normal bulk. If you find it necessary, work your way up to a big bulk. If you're all of the above but worry you might be too old, especially if you're over 30, you can do the same. Start with a normal bulk, and increase only if necessary. Of course, this goes for anyone who's uncomfortable eating a big bulk. You can start small and work your way up.

It's important to note that big bulkers have to lift heavy, and they have to use the lower body lifts (squat and deadlift). Your quads and other lower body muscle groups make up a majority of your body's muscle mass. If you're only doing upper body work because you only care about your "glamor muscles," then you don't need so many extra calories. Working your legs will allow more muscle to be built and it necessitates the huge surplus. Basically, if you do the big bulk, never skip leg day.

And take note: Some experts dispute the value of a bulk in excess of 1,000 surplus calories per day. I personally disagree, though, for a few reasons. One is simply the track record; great strength training coaches have recommended it for decades, and have had success with innumerable athletes. I also know from reading the stories of other hardgainers that some young men struggle for years to gain any muscle until they finally try a big bulk and are able to kickstart their transformation.

In fact, the coaches at Bony to Beastly (who specialize in coaching skinny hardgainers) have found that many of their clients will struggle to gain weight *even after* adding 1,000 kcal. How can it be that you'd weigh a certain amount, add a 1,000-kcal surplus, and still weigh the same? It's because, as these coaches discovered, the metabolisms of hardgainers simply kick into high gear when they start eating more. (Duquette, 2020) Therefore, for some guys, you'll have to eat incredible amounts of food to overcome your unusual calorie-burning abilities.

Finally, I did a big bulk myself, so I know its value from experience. I saw how eating big can make your strength and muscular size explode like nothing else. But because there is limited research on big bulks, we have to combine science here with close observation. Big bulks clearly work best for some, but not for others.

An Easy Shortcut: Watch Your Waist Size and Bodyfat

Fellas, to know quickly whether you've gained too much fat, monitor your waist size. According to strength coach and founder of Barbell Logic Matt Reynolds, shorter guys with a waist from 32 to 36 inches, or taller guys with a waist from 35 to 38 inches, can continue safely bulking. For any male whose waist exceeds 40 inches, you've gained too much weight and should reduce calories (McKay, 2020)

In case those numbers scare you, you should know that it takes a hardgainer a very long time to go from a 32" waist to 40". Chances are, you'll never get even close. Personally, it took me an entire year of eating big to add just three inches to my waist, from 32" to 35". (By the way, my waist eventually dropped down to 31" after I did a cut.).

Your bodyfat should likewise never get into obese levels (25% or more). Some fitness pros will tell you to never exceed 15% bodyfat, while others will tell you the 15-25% bodyfat range is acceptable when it's only temporary for the sake of building muscle. It ultimately depends on the person, and it's something you should discuss with your doctor. Once you get into the unhealthy zone, you need drop the bodyfat with a cut or by training with maintenance calories.

To reiterate, when a young beginner starts a big bulk, he should "fill out" his body within about two months. Once he has a normal bodyweight, that will be the time to start reducing calories so that he can continue bulking but with less fat gain.

Track your progress as described in the previous section. Combine your strength progress numbers with your weight, waist size, bodyfat percent, how comfortable you are with the change to your appearance, and you have all the information you need to adjust your calories and training.

Homework for the Hardgainers

Here's two articles I recommend all hardgainers read before beginning a big bulk:

- "To Be A Beast," by Jordan Feigenbaum (barbellmedicine.com/blog/584-2/)
- "A Clarification," by Mark Rippetoe (startingstrength.com/article/a_clarification)

Choose Your Own Adventure

"Success isn't always about greatness. It's about consistency.
Consistent hard work gains success. Greatness will come."
—Dwayne "The Rock" Johnson

"Motivation is what gets you started. Habit is what keeps you going."
—Jim Ryun, Olympic medalist

If you ask around at the gym, Billy Barbell will tell you, "You gotta eat big to get big, bro." He means eat everything in sight until you're shaped like an upside-down power plug, because he assumes that his goal of getting as strong as humanly possible is everyone else's goal too. The fella over on the elliptical might tell you, "Bulking will make you look like the Hulk; best to stick to cardio and light weights." Then he'll go eat a kale salad with no protein.

I understand both viewpoints, and both are valid if they match your goals. Lots of fat gain can be very demotivating and can take forever to cut later. On the other hand, slow progress can be a killer. But either can be appropriate, depending on who you are.

After a few months to a couple years (depending if you have to add a cut or recomp before you bulk), you'll transition from a beginner to an intermediate. By this point, you'll be a lot stronger, with a lot more muscle, and that much closer to reaching your genetic potential. Your strength gains will have slowed or completely stopped, because your body isn't responding to the training anymore, or you can't recover from your workouts. At this point, you might need a whole new training program, or you might simply need to make tweaks to your current one.

Now you have a lot of options and your goals will determine what you choose. Want to get even stronger? Keep bulking, change your workout routine, and cut the fat later. Some people spend several years going through cycles of bulking and cutting.

Want to quickly get even leaner and ripped? Cut the fat on a deficit while you maintain your muscle.

Want to simply keep the new body you've built? Shift your diet and training to maintenance. Your appearance and body composition will continue to slowly improve.

Want to switch to an activity with more endurance, maybe to run a 5K, rock climb, or learn Muay Thai? Start training for it. You've put on a good base of strength that will make you better at all kinds of activities. You can still strength train in moderation to keep the muscle. In fact, a 2011 study out of the University of Alabama at Birmingham found that you can train as little as once per week and keep most of your muscle (and potentially gain more). (Matthews, How to Maintain Muscle and Strength with Minimal Exercise)

Keep in mind, strength training doesn't necessarily mean weightlifting. Weighted bodyweight movements are plenty, if you know what you're doing. This should be great news for anyone that prefers to work out at home. Once you've put on a good base of muscle and strength, you can potentially keep all of those gains for decades without ever stepping foot in another gym.

Whatever path you choose, *do what keeps you motivated*. It's the only way to stay consistent with workouts. If you like getting strong but you're sick of lifting weights, find something else. Curious about CrossFit? Go try it! Don't want to spend so much time in the gym? Try an at-home routine. You can even build your own gym and work out with friends.

As long as you're healthy and happy with how you look, just do stuff you enjoy.

Chapter 8 Recap

The "big bulk" is only for young (under 35), tall, skinny hardgainers. These are the guys that have the hardest time gaining weight. You'll eat 700 to 1,000 extra calories or more per day. You have to be careful because you can gain weight very fast. Keep in mind, rapid weight gain might be a good thing, even if it means temporarily gaining as much fat as muscle. This bulk should not last more than a few months after which time you can continue bulking but with a smaller caloric surplus. Add 200 extra calories per week until you reach your target surplus.

How fast you can expect to gain weight depends on how fast you can gain muscle. At best, you can gain two to four pounds of muscle per month for the first three months. That would mean potentially gaining four to eight pounds of total bodyweight per month. Your rate of muscle gain will slow over time. After a few years of training, the best you can do is gain a few pounds of muscle per year.

To determine if you're eating the right amount, watch your rate of weight gain and whether your lifts are improving. Also, watch your waist size. At some point, adding more calories won't help, so be careful. If you are closer to skinny-fat than skinny, consider starting with a normal bulk and only add more calories if necessary.

Some experts dispute the value of a big 1,000 calorie bulk, but I believe the track record of coaches as well as my own experience prove otherwise. To learn more about bigtime bulking, read the two articles I recommend. Ultimately, it's up to you how much and how fast you want to grow. After a few months of bulking, you'll have a lot of options for what to do next with your diet and training. Whatever you choose, do what you enjoy.

CHAPTER 9: BULKING HACKS

Plenty of authors will tell you what an ideal bulk looks like: get all of your calories from whole foods, eat tons of vegetables and lean meats, cut sugar completely, etc. When you see that, you know the author never had to eat 5,000+ kcal per day (like I did). When you live it, you realize quickly that you need to cut some corners to get all of those calories in. "Ideal" won't work.

Need to cram in tons of calories and want to get even more out of your bulks? Try these common tips for hardgainers and anyone else who struggles to over-eat.

Eat Calorie-Dense Foods

The smaller your stomach and appetite, the less you should waste precious stomach space on lighter, low-calorie foods like salad, vegetables, and bread. Instead focus on calorie-dense whole foods, healthy foods that pack in as many calories in as few bites as possible. Use the labels on cans and bags to find the most calorie-dense stuff, or search online for more recommendations. Here are examples of some of the most popular high-calorie whole foods bulkers love:

- Healthy oils (e.g. olive oil)
- Nuts and nut butters
- Protein powder
- Dark chocolate
- Fatty red meat
- Ground meat
- Whole milk
- Dried fruit
- White rice
- Fatty fish
- Trail mix

- Avocado
- Bananas
- Granola
- Cheese
- Honey
- Pasta
- Oats

Eat Less-Filling Foods

Foods are more filling when they have more protein, fiber, or water content. What I'm not going to tell you is to stop eating things with protein and fiber, obviously. Instead, you can find workarounds.

One method is to focus on high-calorie options when eating things with protein. If you're going to be eating chicken, for example, have the chicken thigh instead of breast. The thigh has more fat, so you'll eat the same volume of food but get more calories in. To avoid fiber, opt for white carbs instead of brown, and have more fruit than vegetables.

When you can, avoid foods that contain lots of water. For example, have dried fruit instead of regular fruit. A handful of raisins is a lot less filling than an entire bowl of grapes. If you want real fruit, have some more calorie-dense options. For example, you can eat a banana a lot faster than an apple.

Of course, the best method to avoid being overly full is to drink more calories (More on that in a minute.). If you feel the need to have a drink with your meals, consider substituting a high-calorie drink like milk or fruit juice for water. That way, you're at least getting in some calories. Otherwise, it's best to not have any drink as you eat. Water has no calories and will only fill you up faster.

Eat Like It's Your Job

Don't eat three giant meals per day; eat four or five normal-size meals. This way, you'll never have to eat to the point of feeling sick. Or, eat three normal-sized meals with lots of snacks and shakes in between meals. Keep snacks on you—in your car, in your backpack, or at your desk. Anytime you feel like you can eat, eat! Don't wait for your next scheduled meal. If you end up eating more than planned that day, that's a good thing! You can always eat less than planned the next day. For now, you need to think of food as fuel for your body, and eating is your job.

Never Skip Breakfast

If you do, you'll be playing catch up all day. Consider *getting the majority of your calories in by lunch*. There's less pressure to meet your goals the rest of the day. It also helps to *eat right before bedtime*. Your stomach is empty by morning and you avoid ever feeling overly full during the day.

General dieting advice is to avoid slow-digesting food before bed, so that your stomach can rest as you sleep. With bulking, on the other hand, you might benefit from doing just the opposite. Eating slow-digesting calories for dinner will help continue protein-synthesis as you sleep. This includes high-fat foods (e.g. beef and pork), casein protein (perhaps in a shake), and complex carbs (e.g. vegetables and whole grains).

Eat and Drink *Fast*

Don't nibble at your meals; inhale them! When we eat at a normal pace, our stomach gets full and our body signals for us to stop before we've finished our bulk calories. This happens via stretch receptors in the stomach and the release of hormonal signals. (MacDonald 2010) When you eat fast, you get all the calories in before your stomach starts signaling that it's time to stop.

One way to help this is to eat foods that are easier to chew. Eat hamburger instead of steak, or smoke or stew your meat so that it falls off the bone. Crockpots are perfect for this. A big bowl of chili can be consumed a lot faster than can a big plate of fajita steak. Also, have your steak medium instead of rare. The same goes for vegetables. A cooked carrot is softer and easier to chew than a raw one.

Your best bet for getting in enough vegetables without being overly full is to blend them up. At the very least, you can add a handful of spinach to your protein shakes. Not only will these methods help you eat faster, as a bonus, you won't have to chew as much.

Don't Add All Your Surplus Calories on Day 1

The larger your surplus, the more you need to ramp up the calories over the first few weeks. This will give your body time to adjust to the increase in consumption. You can still begin your workouts as you ramp up the food intake. You'll gain strength and mass, which will kick into high gear once you're eating your full surplus.

If you instead decide to eat all of you new calories from the first day, you'll run into some issues: your stomach hasn't expanded yet to accommodate higher food intake, so you'll feel sick when you overeat; you'll get lethargic after a giant meal because your body isn't yet adapted to processing so much energy; those giant meals might make you bloated, gassy, and give you serious acid reflux.

Make Your Food Taste Good

Add spices, sauces and condiments, and use different techniques like grilling and baking. Eating lots of healthy food will be gross if your meals are bland. (Personally, I once ate canned salmon heated in a microwave, with nothing added to it. Don't do what I did; you can't un-taste it.) This is why so many people complain that healthy food is "boring." It's because they aren't taking the time to make it taste better.

Stay Hydrated

Staying hydrated actually makes you hungrier, so drink lots of water (just not right before or during a meal, when of course you want your stomach to be as empty as possible). A general recommendation is to drink half your body weight in fluid ounces of water per day. If drinking that much is filling you up and preventing you from eating enough, then drink less. Keep in mind, food itself has lots of water content.

Buy a large reusable bottle and take it everywhere you go. Consider adding electrolytes to your water, especially during workouts. They come in either tablet or liquid form, and can be purchased online and at nutrition stores. Simple table salt is also a natural electrolyte.

Improve Your Digestion

Everything will go down easier and you'll have less intestinal distress when you can digest more efficiently. Probiotics are a beneficial bacteria you can eat which aid digestion. They're found in fermented foods like kimchi and sauerkraut and yogurts with live and active cultures. Or, take them in pill-form.

Also, be sure to chew your food well before swallowing, which will help your body absorb more nutrients. It also helps to reduce stress as much as possible, as stress is linked to stomach ulcers, diarrhea, constipation, and IBS.

Other supplements that have been linked to a healthy gut: glutamine (found in eggs, turkey, and almonds), zinc (high in shellfish, beef, and sunflower seeds), l-glutamine, and ginger.

Don't Do Things That Are Known to Reduce Your Appetite

This part's self-explanatory. Don't make things harder than they have to be. Cut out smoking, recreational drugs, fiber supplements (you should be getting plenty of fiber from your diet), and other items that will make you less hungry.

Avoid Stress

Similar to the last point, stress can negatively affect your appetite. This is especially true for folks who don't instinctively turn to food for comfort. Some people get stressed or depressed and turn to comfort food, like eating a tub of ice cream after a break up. This is why some people put on weight when put in stressful situations (see "the freshmen 15") or when life just gets hard. It's emotional eating, and it's totally understandable.

However, naturally skinny guys tend to find other outlets for stress, not food. While others might sit in bed with a bag of chocolates after a hard day, hardgainers are more likely to forget to eat altogether.

How you address your stress depends on what's causing it. Sometimes the fix can be as simple as going for a walk, talking to a friend, or just taking a quick break from a busy life to sit and watch a movie. Some problems are deeper, though, and your solution might be very personal and specific, from addressing emotional issues to grappling with a guilty conscience. My two cents: prayer and reading Scripture have helped me tremendously during hard times.

As far as physical solutions, getting lots of sleep and consistently working out are both known to reduce stress. Companies know this, and it's why they'll often encourage employees to take breaks and move around during the workday. Sleep is no joke, either. According to the American Psychological Association, even slight sleep deprivation can affect your memory, judgement, and mood. They also found that most Americans would be happier and healthier with an extra 60 to 90 minutes of sleep each night. (Stress and Sleep, 2013)

Drink Your Calories

Protein shakes and "mass gainer" shakes are quick and easy to make, you can take them on-the-go to work or class, and you can squeeze in a thousand calories or more in a single glass, very difficult to achieve with solid food meals. They also digest faster than solids, so you don't feel full as long and you can eat more again sooner. Shakes are essential for hard-gainers. Throw in some peanut butter or olive oil to add some serious calories. It's important to have variety in your diet, but you can still have multiple shakes per day, especially when you add variety to the shakes themselves: fruit, vegetables, nuts, oats, healthy oils, protein powder, etc.

Weight gainers found at stores are usually filled with sugar and other unhealthy crap, so consider making your own with a blender. Also, don't sip on it for an hour. *Chug it quickly!* If your calorie target is 4,000 per day and you have a 1,000 calorie shake for breakfast, that's a quarter of your required calories over in a couple minutes.

GOMAD ("Gallon of Milk A Day")

If a shake is too much, simply drink whole milk. Consider having a glass with every single meal. Some hardgainers, including myself, have found success drinking an entire gallon of whole milk per day. It can help put on those first 20+ pounds if you start off underweight.

One gallon of whole milk contains 1,200 kcal with 96g of carbs and 64g of both protein and fat. That's a pretty excellent mix of macros. If you spread out your consumption of the entire gallon throughout the day, you're guaranteed to have a good flow of protein all day, every day. Many guys who use GOMAD will simply eat three normal meals a day while drinking the milk in between meals.

Please note that GOMAD is only for young, underweight men who struggle adding mass with food alone, and shouldn't be done longer than six to eight weeks. Some guys do it for longer, but it's controversial. Mark Rippetoe's free online article "A Clarification" (startingstrength.com/article/a_clarification) can help you decide if GOMAD is right for you.

Track Your Food Intake to Make Sure You're Really Eating as Much as You Think

This is a big one. It's easy to overestimate your calorie intake, and it might be why you're not gaining. Weigh and measure your food if necessary, and consider a food tracking app. I've found it helps to sit down and figure out how many calories are in the main foods you eat. That way you don't have to constantly check nutrition labels. You'll already know exactly what's in that bowl of oatmeal or that PB&J. Speaking of...

Peanut Butter and Jelly Sandwiches Are the Perfect Snack for Bulkers

Tons of fat and protein, cheap, easy to make, and you can take them on the go. Use whole grain bread and "natural" peanut butter with a healthier oil for a "cleaner" sandwich. Consider sitting down on your prep day and using an entire loaf of bread to make a dozen sandwiches at once. Leave them in the refrigerator and eat them throughout the week.

Add Olive Oil (Or Other Healthy Oils) To Everything

In your shakes, on your meals, or even alone in a shot glass for instant calories. Sound gross? Maybe, but it's a lot easier than eating another entire meal. You don't want to get the majority of your calories from oil, or any other single source, and I'm not saying to have five shots of EVOO every day. You will probably benefit from more oil than you're used to, though.

Chapter 9 Recap

Eat calorie dense foods so you don't have to eat as much overall; eat like it's your job (i.e. eat constantly); never skip breakfast (or dinner) so your stomach is rarely empty; eat and drink fast before your body knows what hit it; slowly ramp up the caloric surplus to give your body time to adjust; take the time to cook your food and make it taste good; stay hydrated and get plenty of electrolytes for your training; don't do things that reduce your appetite like smoking; drink your calories with healthy, calorie-dense ingredients; consider GOMAD if you're a hardgainer; track your calories to make sure you're eating enough; make PB&J sandwiches your friend; add healthy oils like olive oil to everything.

CHAPTER 10: CUTTING THE FAT

Let's say you're six months into your bulk. Your strength has skyrocketed and you've gained maybe twenty or thirty pounds. Most of it is muscle, but some was fat, enough that you're starting to look a little "fluffy." You want to get rid of the new fat gains, so now is finally the time to perform a "cut." The purpose of cutting is to lose fat, and to do so quickly, you'll need to lose weight. Which means eating a calorie deficit.

Before discussing cutting, I'll quickly mention another option for dropping bodyfat, and that's performing a "recomp," short for "body recomposition." This means eating maintenance calories while you continue to strength train. When you do this, you'll reduce your bodyfat percentage and probably build some muscle in the process. You'll stay around the same weight, but your ratio of muscle to fat will improve significantly. I'll go into further detail later about how to train while in maintenance mode.

Some guys prefer recomping to cutting because they're basically happy with how they look, so they're okay with getting leaner more slowly. Still, there are downsides to recomping. Eating your exact maintenance calories is a tightrope walk, and it's very easy to go over or under. Your top priority will be to hit your calorie target as closely as possible each day. Also, the key word about recomping is *slow*. A recomp can take up to several months before you're at your desired bodyfat level, but it depends on how high your bodyfat level is to begin with. Most guys would rather get there faster, and that's where cutting comes in.

The downside to cutting is twofold: you probably won't build much muscle while you do it, unless you're obese or overly-fat to start with. Although, some people can, even well-trained athletes with healthy bodyfat. A 2011 study showed that athletes who lost 0.7% of bodyweight (roughly 1-1.5lbs) per week were able to build muscle at the same time. (Garthe, 2011)

The other concern with cutting: You can actively lose muscle as you lose weight. If you cut too fast, or without proper diet and training, your body might begin burning muscle and not just bodyfat. To keep your muscle, you'll continue working out with heavy weights doing whole-body, compound movements (but more on this in later chapters). This means the purpose of your training will now be to at least maintain muscle, not necessarily build it.

The upside to cutting is you can reduce your training volume and frequency significantly, similar to training on a recomp. Thankfully, it's much easier to maintain muscle than it is to build it. You also might add a few hours of cardio each week to speed up the fat loss. The more trained you are, the more intense your cardio can be.

The more aggressively you cut (i.e. the less food you eat), the faster you'll lose weight and burn fat. However, cut too aggressively and you'll lose muscle; not aggressively enough and your cutting period will last too long. Restricting calories isn't easy, so you don't want your cut to last longer than it has to.

Who Should Cut?

1. *Are you overweight (BMI over 30) or at an obese bodyfat level (25% or greater)?* In either case, you should cut, or recomp at the very least.
2. *Are you at a normal weight but your BF% is too high?* You can either cut to lose fat quickly or eat maintenance calories while you recomp and lose it slowly.
3. *Do you have a healthy amount of body fat but you want to be even leaner (while still being in a healthy bodyfat range)?* Same: cut or recomp.
4. *Do you want to get bigger and stronger quickly?* Keep bulking.
5. *Are you still underweight or have a very low BF% number?* Absolutely keep bulking.

How Long Will the Cut Last?

A typical answer is two to four months, but it depends on what your current bodyfat percentage is, how much fat you want to lose, and how aggressively you want to cut. As long as you get down to the healthy BF% range, and don't drop below that healthy range, you can stop the cut at any time. The healthy bodyfat range is typically 8 to 15%, but there's wiggle room on either side, and it depends on the individual. However you choose to cut, be patient and don't lose that hard-gained muscle mass; or even worse, make yourself sick.

The more bodyfat you have to start, the quicker you'll burn it. If, for example, you wanted to drop three percentage points from 18% to 15%, that might take six weeks or less of aggressive cutting. However, if you wanted to drop three points from 13% to 10%, that would take much longer. This is because it's harder to lose fat when you're already lean. Likewise, the more fat you want to lose, the longer it will take. A cut that will drop you five percentage points, say from 15% to 10%, could take a few months.

Many guys prefer to cut down fat enough to get a ripped and sculpted look. That's about 8 to 12% in men. The younger or more naturally lean you are, the easier it will be to get down to these levels. Keep in mind that you might not have a ton of muscle yet (or at least not your "ideal" amount), so the way you'll look at say 10% bodyfat won't be the same as someone who's extremely muscular at 10%. This is why you might decide to keep bulking.

These cycles of bulking and cutting can sometimes last an entire adult life. Some people prefer to bulk during fall and winter (often referred to by them as "bulking season"), because they can hide the temporary fat gain under their winter clothes. Then they'll cut in time for spring and summer (aka "bathing suit season").

Take note: anytime you transition from a cut to a bulk, or from maintenance calories to a bulk, ease into it. Just like the first time you bulked, add in the surplus slowly over the first few weeks until you're at the full bulk.

How Fast Should I Lose Fat During a Cut?

The bigger the calorie deficit, the faster you'll cut fat. Sometimes faster is better. In fact, a 2015 study by scientists at the University of Jyväskylä in Finland showed that reducing calories by 25% led to four times the fat loss than a 10% reduction, with no difference in muscle loss. (Legge, n.d.)

As part of a 2011 study of weight-loss in athletes, the researchers claimed that while athletes on a cut are advised to lose up to 2.2lbs per week (roughly 1.4% of bodyweight), a loss of 1.1lb weekly (roughly 0.7% of bodyweight) is better for preserving lean mass and athletic performance. (Garthe et al., 2011)

It's generally agreed that you can lose no more than a maximum of 2 pounds of body weight per week without losing muscle, but it depends on your weight. If you weigh under 200 pounds, that number might be even lower. In that case, shoot for a weekly loss of 0.5 to 1% of bodyweight. So if you weigh 175 pounds, you'd lose around 0.9 to 1.75 pounds per week.

For more precision, consider the following method. According to Greg Nuckols, cutting should be based on the following formula (Nuckols, 2017):

Bodyfat percentage divided by 20 = percentage of your current bodyweight you should lose per week.

So, if you're 20% bodyfat, you'd lose 1% of bodyweight per week (0.2/20 = 0.01, or 1%). A 180-pound man would lose 1.8 pounds per week. At 10% bodyfat, you'd lose 0.5% of bodyweight per week (0.1/20 = 0.005, or 0.5%). At 180 pounds, you'd lose 0.9 pounds per week.

This way, the higher your bodyfat is, the more aggressively you'll cut. The only guys who would exceed a loss of two pounds per week are those who are heavy (200+) and have a very high BF%. So a guy weighing 200 pounds at 25% BF would lose 2.5 pounds per week.

Keep in mind, as you lose weight, the formula will stay the same but your rate of weight loss will slowly drop. For example, if the 200-pound guy with 25% BF followed the above formula and lost 2.5 pounds per week, in two months he would drop to 180 pounds and say 18% BF. If he plugged his new numbers into the formula, it would tell him to now lose 1.6 pounds per week (0.18/20 = 0.009; 0.9% of 180 = 1.6).

Again, you don't have to get that precise. If you don't feel like doing all of that math, just shoot for weight loss of two pounds per week (for bigger guys) or one pound per week (for smaller guys).

By the way, you might want to take a few days to recalculate your maintenance calories. They've likely increased since you've added more muscle mass, which burns more calories than bodyfat.

Your Fat Loss Will Slow Down

Over time, your body will naturally adjust to the calorie deficit. Because of this, you will continue losing fat but at a slower rate. According to strength coach and founder of Barbell Medicine Dr. Jordan Feigenbaum, after being in a caloric deficit for a while, "as an adaptive process, the body slows down many calorie-burning processes to preserve homeostasis. We predict that the rate of weight loss will decrease as this occurs." Once you increase the calories back to a normal level, your "metabolism should increase back to previous levels." (Feigenbaum, 2015)

Therefore, once you hit that wall of slower fat loss, you'll have to reduce calories even more to keep losing weight at a significant rate (if that's what you prefer). But it's a temporary change and will not "destroy your metabolism" as some think.

Should I Cut Before Bulking?

A hypothetical: Let's say 30-year-old Jacob is a 6-foot-tall 180-pound man with 18% body fat. He's also a beginner. He's not overweight but he does have excess fat (a typical skinny-fat scenario). He's worried that if he bulks up, he'll quickly enter obese territory with his bodyfat. As you'll recall, in this situation, I recommend doing a "recomp" for a few months, then bulking. Instead, he decides to make an even quicker change by cutting first.

An aggressive cut, lasting six weeks, brings Jacob down from 180 to 170 pounds and from 18% to 13% body fat. He lost 10 pounds and 5% bodyfat. He didn't lose any muscle, but he didn't have much to begin with. At this point, he'll be leaner, but he'll also look weaker, with just a little flab hanging over virtually nothing but bone. Sure, he's lean now, but he isn't exactly "healthy."

On the other hand, let's say he decided instead to bulk up from the get-go using a small bulk, gaining around a half pound per week and keeping fat gain to a minimum. After five months, he went from 180 to 190 pounds and from 18 to 23% bodyfat. He gained 10 pounds (maybe 6 or 7 pounds of muscle) and an additional 5% bodyfat. He's not at an ideal bodyfat percentage, and there are risks involved, but he's not obese. In the mirror, he sees a guy who's more filled-out and a whole lot stronger. He's not really "jacked" yet, but for the first time in his life, he's not scrawny.

Question: Was the original scenario of cutting first worth it? Or should Jacob have just bulked up? Should he have done neither and instead followed my advice to recomp, then bulk? Everyone's answer will be different.

The downside to bulking first: He gained more fat than is ideal, and it's potentially risky. Many fitness pros will tell you that a man should bulk up only when his bodyfat is 15% or below. (Others will say that even bulking in the 15-25% range is fine for a while.) Even if the fat gain isn't dangerous for Jacob, he's having to use a small bulk due to both his age and his already high bodyfat, so his muscle gains are quite slow.

The downside to cutting first: Others will tell you it's crazy to lose weight when you have no muscle to begin with. You'll only look scrawnier, you'll be even weaker, and you'll potentially lose what little muscle you have. Still, his cut took only six weeks, which meant he could begin bulking up sooner than if he had recomped instead.

My personal view is that recomping is a nice middle ground in this situation: you never get smaller than you are to start, you only get leaner, and you can build a little muscle while you're at it. With a five-month recomp, Jacob would have gained a decent amount of muscle (and a ton of strength) and gotten very lean. He would then have the option to bulk up for faster gains. Still, recomping has a downside, too: it's slow progress and it might take several months before you can begin bulking.

To bring it all back to my original question that bulkers commonly ask — "Should I cut before I bulk?" — I think it's usually best to "recomp." But there are pros and cons to each choice. Ultimately, it's up to you.

How Much Should I Eat During a Cut?

We've covered how quickly you should lose weight. Now I'll explain a couple options for how to pick your calories so you can achieve that rate of weight loss.

A common recommendation to start a cut is to *reduce your calorie intake by 20 to 25% of your maintenance calories*. This might come out to a reduction of around 500 kcal, which itself is a very typical recommendation for fat loss. According to the Mayo Clinic, as a general rule, cutting by 500-1,000 kcal a day will lead to a loss of 1-2lbs per week. (Counting calories: Get back to weight-loss basics, 2020 Therefore, for a bigger guy who wants to lose 2lbs per week, you'll likely need to eat even fewer than 25% of maintenance calories.

Whether you're shooting for a loss of 1 pound per week (smaller guys) or 2 pounds per week (bigger guys), or if you're basing it on coach Nuckols' formula. Add or subtract calories accordingly to lose at your desired rate of weight loss.

What Should I Eat During a Cut?

You should eat essentially the same foods and macros as you would while bulking. The same goes for eating maintenance calories on a recomp. You should still eat mostly whole foods (at least 80% clean foods being a good target) and get plenty of protein. Fitness pros generally recommend upping the protein during a cut, so that you might have up to two grams per pound of bodyweight. This has two main benefits: you make sure you don't lose an ounce of muscle due to a lack of protein, and you end up eating less carbs and fat (which contains more calories per gram).

Since you're trying to lose (or maintain) weight, cutting carbs will likely help. You'll still benefit from them to fuel your workouts, so if you choose to go low-carb, try to get most of your carb intake right before, during, or after your workouts. You might cut them completely on off days.

When to Stop Cutting

You might get tempted to take your cut too far. It can be pretty exciting to see yourself get more and more shredded. Still, you need to stay healthy and not put yourself in harm's way. As your bodyfat drops to very low levels, you can start running into serious problems. Here are some red flags that it's time to stop cutting:

- Depression, irritation, mood swings, and malaise
- Loss of motivation, whether fitness-related or general burnout
- Worse gym performance: low energy, failing reps, less strength

- Signs of nutrient deficiency: hair loss, weakened immune system, fatigue
- When you hit multiple weight loss "plateaus" and you're forced to eat less and less to keep losing weight.

Tips to Make Your Cut Easier

Like bulking, losing weight is hard. It takes dedication and discipline. The hardest part is dealing with hunger. Here are a few tips to help you stick to your cut and to get it over with as soon as possible:

- *Continue lifting heavy.* You need to do this anyways in order to preserve muscle, but it's worth noting that lifting heavy weights is an excellent way to burn energy.
- *High-intensity interval training (HIIT).* These are intense cardio exercises that will get your heart racing and expend tons of energy. It's perfect for intermediates, but not ideal if you're a totally out-of-shape beginner. It includes biking, elliptical, rowing, jump rope, running, and swimming. HIIT is quick and efficient (perfect for guys with busy lives). HIIT involves doing repetitions of strenuous cardio exercises. Or you might do a circuit of bodyweight exercises in rapid succession. So you might do 30 seconds of pushups, then a quick rest, 30 seconds of kettlebell goblet squats, rest, 30 seconds of pull ups, rest, and so on.
- *Low-intensity steady-state (LISS).* This is a light and easy cardio routine that's perfect for novices who are very out of shape. It can be as simple as walking first thing in the morning (perhaps fasted and with coffee) five times per week.
- *Sprint, don't jog.* If you prefer to run for your cardio, consider doing sprints instead, even hill sprints. Similar to HIIT, you'll burn more calories in less time. Again, this isn't ideal for total beginners as it can cut into your training recovery.
- *Eat more filling food.* When you're trying to lose or maintain weight, feeling full is a good thing. Unlike with a bulk, you shouldn't avoid foods that make you feel full: high-protein (even when it's low-fat), high-fiber, and high-water content. If you aren't getting enough fiber from your diet, consider taking it in powder or pill form.

- *Only eat when you're hungry.* When you bulk, it's good to graze throughout the day. When cutting, it's better to eat less often and experience some hunger-pains.
- *Drink more water.* It might seem like a paradox that drinking water would help with both gaining weight and losing weight. Yet bodybuilders clearly benefit from staying well-hydrated when they cut.
- *Avoid unnecessary calories.* You can still have your favorite junk food in moderation, but it's best to avoid high-sugar, high-fat, greasy-carb calories as much as possible. Try substituting your favorite bulking snacks with lower-calorie options. Add vinaigrettes to your salads instead of oils, add water to your protein shakes instead of milk, and so on.
- *Drink caffeine.* Caffeine is both a natural nootropic (i.e. a mental booster) and great way to stay focused and energized. Sometimes it takes focusing on everyday tasks in life to deal with the background problem of hunger. Your workouts will benefit from it too.
- *Track your calories.* It will be incredibly tempting to eat more than your allotted calories for the day, and tracking your exact intake will help keep you honest.
- *Avoid liquid carbs.* Sugary sports drinks, non-diet sodas, and carb-heavy shakes should be avoided.
- *Intermittent fasting.* This is where you limit all of your eating for the day to a shortened window of time. It can be as simple as skipping breakfast every morning.
- *Use little tricks to reduce meal portions and appetite.* Some common tricks include drinking a glass of water before eating; When you eat, take a bite, put your fork down, chew and swallow, take another bite, repeat (you'll end up eating less); Brush your teeth right after dinner; Chew gum to stave off hunger (there's actually science behind this).

Take note: If you're a total beginner (aka rank novice) and you're "recomping" to lose fat, don't go too hard on the HIIT and cardio. An intermediate can probably get away with intense cardio like sprints or very strenuous forms of HIIT several times per week. A true beginner, on the other hand, shouldn't go so hard (as there's a risk of overtraining). Dr. Feigenbaum would suggest doing moderate HIIT with something like a prowler or rower machine. Since your strength training is still fairly easy (as you're in the very early stages), even moderate cardio or HIIT is helpful. It will tend to help your workout recovery, increase your metabolic rate, and improve your cardiorespiratory capacity. Feigenbaum suggests starting with two days of HIIT per week, and potentially adding a third day if tolerable. These HIIT sessions can be done on off days. (Feigenbaum, 2015)

Chapter 10 Recap

After bulking for a while, you might want to cut some of the bodyfat to get lean. You have to be careful when cutting because you don't want to lose muscle. The more aggressive you cut (i.e. the larger a caloric deficit you use), the faster you'll lose weight.

You should cut if you're overweight, your bodyfat percent is too high, or you want to get leaner while staying in a healthy bodyfat range. An aggressive cut might last several weeks if you want to get down to the lower bodyfat levels. You can go through cycles of bulking and cutting throughout your lifetime and you can choose specific "seasons" for when to do this.

When you cut, your body will slowly adjust to the lower calories and you'll have to eat even less in order to keep losing weight. Fortunately, your metabolism will adjust back to normal once the cut ends.

It's up to you if you want to cut before you ever start bulking, but it's generally a better idea to recomp first, then bulk up.

Simply reduce calories by 20 to 25% of your maintenance calories. Bigger guys should aim to lose about two pounds per week, while smaller guys should aim to lose more like one pound per week. Adjust calories accordingly.

Continue eating mostly whole foods and lots of protein. Adjust carb intake as necessary for better weight loss and maintenance. And consider the common tips I've provided for cutting successfully and quickly.

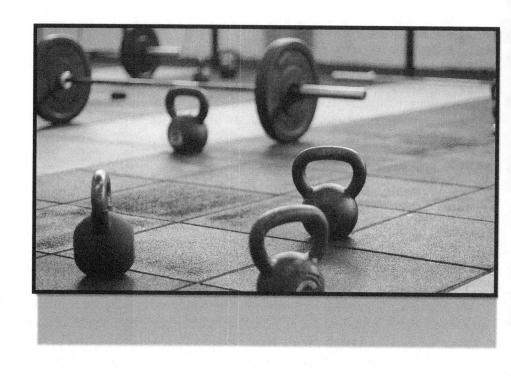

PART 3: STRENGTH TRAINING

CHAPTER 11: WHY STRENGTH TRAINING?

"No citizen has a right to be an amateur in the matter of physical training...what a disgrace it is for a man to grow old without ever seeing the beauty and strength of which his body is capable."
—Socrates

"If you think lifting is dangerous, try being weak. Being weak is dangerous."
—Bret Contreras, sports scientist

Now that we've covered how to bulk up with your diet, there's one more thing needed to transform your body—strength training. It's also called "resistance training" because you'll be using an external resistance, like dumbbells, barbells or tension cables, to contract and grow your muscles. From here on, I might refer to all of these things as "lifting" or "training."

As I discussed in an earlier chapter, the whole reason to bulk up is to have the extra calories needed to build muscle. If your body is a car, and bulking is the fuel, then training is the actual road trip. Without training, your tank will be full but the car will just be sitting idle (i.e. laying around the couch getting fat).

I know strength training sounds intimidating. I was hesitant to try it myself. To my surprise, I was hooked within the first week or two. As soon as you get into the groove of following a training program—and you'll get into the groove quickly—it feels normal. You'll soon realize you were afraid of a boogeyman.

It's also worth the effort, and not just because you'll look better. Here are just a few of the benefits to training and building muscle (Iliades, 2019) (7 Body and Mind Benefits of Building Muscle, n.d.) (Fetters, 2018):

- Improved mood, energy, and sleep
- Clearer thinking with less anxiety and depression
- Faster metabolism (you'll burn fat easier) and greater insulin sensitivity
- Healthier heart with improved blood pressure and blood-sugar level
- Better balance and less risk of falling
- Stronger bones and less risk of fracture
- More flexibility and less back pain
- Less inflammation and a stronger immune system
- Improvement in a range of illnesses, including arthritis, fibromyalgia, and many more
- Lower risk of disease, longer lifespan, and higher quality of life
- Greater body confidence and better physical appearance
- Greater mental resilience

Will I Look Like One of Those Enormous Bodybuilders?

As we covered earlier, the guys you see in bodybuilding competitions are doing something very different than what you'll be doing. It took those guys years upon years of constant lifting, and often drugs to supplement their intense workouts. In his prime, Arnold Schwarzenegger lifted five hours a day, six days a week, and you will not be training nearly this much. Obviously, I don't recommend drug use either. Anabolic steroids will wreak havoc on your body: reduced sperm count, baldness, shrunken testicles, breast development (yes, in men), severe acne, increased risk of prostate cancer, and more. (Anabolic Steroid Misuse, 2018)

You will certainly get bigger and add some fat when you bulk, but that doesn't mean you'll end up looking bad. Quite the opposite! It's true that if your abs currently have a ripped six-pack look, you will lose this for a while as you gain weight. But as Mark Rippetoe said, "The fact that your abs smooth out a little while your shoulders, chest, legs, and hips get bigger will only be a cause for concern to you. Because you're going to look better to everybody else when you're bigger. I promise." (Rippetoe, Maybe You Should GAIN Weight, 2017)

The point being, you're not going to look particularly fat or roided-up when you bulk, *you're going to look like a man*, and a healthy one at that. If you need further convincing, there are innumerable online polls that show that women tend to prefer men with more normal bodyfat levels vs. men that are extremely shredded. In fact, dropping your bodyfat down from say 12% to 8% isn't going to impress anyone but your gym buddies. As long as you're in a healthy bodyfat range (usually around 15% or lower), you're going to look awesome.

Is Strength Training Safe?

In general: yes, absolutely. The exception is if you already have injuries, mobility issues, or illnesses that can make strength training dangerous. If so, it's imperative that you talk to a doctor before you lift. If you try strength training and experience acute pain, not simply discomfort or soreness, you should also stop immediately and see a doctor.

Research has shown that lifting is very safe compared to other exercises and sports. In fact, you're 6 to 10 times more likely to get hurt playing everyday sports like soccer and basketball than from heavy weightlifting. In fact, if you lift five hours per week, on average you go four years without any injury at all, even minor ones. (Matthews, How Dangerous Is Weightlifting? What 20 Studies Have to Say, n.d.) Not only that, it's safe for nearly everyone—men, women, children, the elderly, the pregnant, and even with some forms of disability.

Like any sport, the longer you lift, the more likely an injury becomes, especially minor problems like tendonitis and joint pain. These tend to turn into "repetitive stress injuries" when you ignore them, so take care to listen to what your body is telling you.

Of course, lifting weights is only safe *when done properly*. You can't start throwing 50-pound dumbbells around on day one. Lifting the appropriate amount and with good form is very important. But we'll look a lot more at this in later chapters, as well as the main types of strength training and the various programs you can try.

A warning about lifting really heavy: it's very common for guys to get into lifting and to get fixates on lifting enormous amounts of weight. This is a fantastic goal, but it can lead to missing the forest for the trees. Once you get really strong (say benching 1.5xbodyweight or squatting 2xbodyweight), getting even stronger after this point won't necessarily make you fitter. There's nothing wrong with wanting to get even bigger and stronger or even to become a competitive powerlifter. Still, it helps to keep a balanced perspective. Ask around at any elite gym and you'll learn that a career of lifting *really heavy* almost always leads to injuries, some irreversible.

This doesn't mean it's impossible to powerlift safely, it's that real life isn't "ideal:" one day you'll have to train when you're sick or sleep-deprived, or your program will call for adding weight to a lift even though your form still needs work, or your program will call for using a lift that has never really felt right to you, and so on. At some point, when you're pushing your body to it's limits, you're likely to make a trade-off that says, "To get more gains, you'll have to take more risks." If your goal is to get super strong, that's awesome. I want you to be stronger and bigger, but also with healthy joints into old age. Just be careful, kings!

But next, let's get down to the nitty gritty about how your training will build muscle. It's important to understand these principles instead of just memorizing a program. I know it's a lot of information, but you do actually need to know it, in order to make smart decisions about what kind of strength training is best for you, how to do it safely, and how to get the most out of your training.

How Muscles Work

Simply put, your muscles are what allow you to move—that is, move against the force of gravity. When you curl a dumbbell, one of your arm muscles (your bicep) contracts, while another nearby muscle (your tricep) elongates, allowing your arm to bend at one of its joints (in this case, the elbow).

Our bodies have hundreds of separate muscles, and each one is made up of millions of fibers that are each the thickness of a hair. Some muscle fibers are "slow twitch," which help with endurance activities like running a marathon. Others are "fast twitch" for short bursts of energy, like sprinting. Everyone has a unique mix of naturally superior slow and fast twitch muscles, which determines the activities we're naturally better at.

It used to be believed that you were stuck with whatever type of muscle tone you were born with. However, recent research suggests you can change that. Just because you're born a long-distance runner doesn't mean you can't learn to be explosive too. (Heffernan, 2020)

To make your body build muscle, you have to "tell it" to do so. If the hardest thing you do on an average day is walk up a few flights of stairs, then your body has no reason to get any stronger than that. You have to do something harder, like climb more steps, steeper steps, or while carrying extra weight. That will tell your body that it needs to grow.

When you train with weights (or even your own bodyweight) in the gym, you're telling your body, "I need you to be stronger so I can lift this weight without struggling." If you eat right and rest enough, your body will respond, "I got you."

Hypertrophy

Strength training increases the size and volume of our muscle fibers and makes them stronger. This is called hypertrophy and there's two kinds: *myofibril hypertrophy* is when the fibers are "traumatized" during a workout, building back up in greater volume and density (making your muscles stronger and slightly larger), while *sarcoplasmic hypertrophy* is when the fibers retain a higher amount of fluid and energy resources post-workout (making your muscles bigger with no increase in strength). (Reid, n.d.) You can alter your lifting routine to favor one type of hypertrophy over the other, or you can focus on both equally.

There's more than one way to experience hypertrophy, and using heavy weights is simply one way to do so. Basically, muscle growth involves more than the heaviness of the actual weights. There's also time under tension, neuromuscular improvements, blood flow, and more. (Cortes, 2020)

Stress, Recover, Adapt

"The pain you feel today will be the strength you feel tomorrow."
— Arnold Schwarzenegger

In the most basic terms, strength training puts stress on your body and slightly damages your muscle fibers. Proper diet and sleep help your body recover and repair those fibers. The result is bigger and stronger muscles. (Physiology of Strength Training: Stress, Recovery, Adaptation., n.d.)

It's like a Texan moving to Alaska. The first few weeks of the bitter cold will be tough. Then they'll adapt to it and be able to handle even colder weather. In the fitness world, this is called "progressive overload." It means doing a little more during this workout than you did last time. Usually this means using heavier and heavier weights, fully recovering each time, and you'll get stronger and stronger. It can also mean using more repetitions (or "reps"), slower reps, less rest time, and so on. Programs focused on getting especially strong will use heavier weight with fewer reps, while programs focused on getting especially big muscles will use higher reps and lower weights.

3 Rules of Recovery

Fun fact: muscle doesn't get built while you work out. It's while you recover after the workout, especially while you sleep. Your body needs rest in order to repair torn muscle tissue, lost glycogen and other body fluids, and even your overstressed nervous system. It's the repairing of these things that makes muscles bigger and stronger. It usually takes about 48 hours to recover from a workout when you're a beginner. Therefore, as a general rule, beginners should work out no more than every other day. As you become an intermediate and you gradually get closer to being advanced, you can recover from workouts faster and faster and can therefore work out more often.

Here are the other three main rules for a fast and safe recovery:

1. *Sleep plenty,* at least eight hours. If you work out and don't sleep well for the next two nights, you might not gain anything. However, it depends on the person. Some guys need more sleep, some less.
2. *Eat enough.* You already know this. Eat consistently too. Every workout requires recovery, which means you must eat enough even on off days (i.e. days you don't work out).
3. *Take it easy* outside of workouts. An intense hike the day after a training session will make recovery harder if not impossible. This is especially true

if you're not eating enough. In fact, even emotional stress can take a toll on recovery.

How Fast Will I See Results?

As you'll recall, it depends how aggressive your training and diet programs are, and your particular factors such as age and how far you are from your genetic potential for muscle gains. Generally, under the best conditions, according to the Lye McDonald model, in your first year of consistent bulking and strength training, you'd gain 20 to 25 pounds of muscle. Your second year more like 10 to 12 pounds of muscle, your third year 5 to 6 pounds of muscle, and 2 to 3 pounds of muscle for all years after that.

Your first few months as a beginner will see the fastest pace of gains, up to two to four pounds of muscle per month. Skinny hardgainers who have very little muscle to start with can potentially gain even faster than that. Once a hardgainer's body fills out with a more typical amount of bodyweight and muscle, their gains will slow to a more average pace.

Regardless of where you start, as you progress from beginner to intermediate to advanced, the gains will come slower and slower, and you'll get closer and closer to fulfilling your genetic potential.

"Newb" Gains

You'll recall that when you're a newbie to strength training, you'll get stronger very quickly *at first*. This is due largely to the fact that your nervous system itself, and not just your muscles, will be getting stronger. As Greg Nuckols explains it, "Your nervous system learns how to use the muscle mass you already have to efficiently perform the movement." (Lee, 2015)

But be warned, these nervous system "gains" will go away after a few weeks to months (potentially up to a year). Everyone eventually hits a wall in their training when their newb gains run out, so don't be discouraged when it happens to you too. You can still build lots of muscle and strength after this point.

Depending on who you ask, "newbie gains" might also refer to the extreme rate of muscle gains that some beginners are capable of. The more underweight you are at the start, the greater potential you have for insane gains.

Chapter 11 Recap

Strength training (aka resistance training) is what allows you to build muscle, and there's a good chance you'll learn to love it. The benefits of strength training include improved emotional state, better sleep, a faster metabolism, a healthier heart, stronger bones, lower risk of a range of diseases, and much more.

Training a few hours per week won't make you look like a bodybuilder, but you will gain some size. You might be doubtful, but you'll probably love the way the extra bodyweight makes you look. Despite what you might have heard, training is very safe when performed properly; safer than most other sports.

Muscles are what allow our bodies to move. You have a mix of "slow twitch" and "fast twitch" muscles, each one making you naturally better at certain activities. Thankfully, you can become better at whichever activity you're not naturally gifted with (i.e. you're not "stuck" with your genetics).

Training "tells" your body to grow and hypertrophy is the result. That means you'll get bigger muscles, stronger muscles, or a mix of both. Training does this by putting a stress on your body that you have to recover from, and proper diet and sleep allow this recovery.

"Progressive overload" means you'll be using heavier and heavier weights (or more reps) over time. To recover from each workout, you need plenty of sleep, calories, and rest. You can expect 1 to 2 pounds of muscle per month at first. Your first few months of training as a beginner will see a faster rate of growth. Eventually these quick gains will dwindle, but you can still bulk and gain.

CHAPTER 12: EVERYTHING YOU NEED TO KNOW ABOUT TRAINING PRINCIPLES

There are entire sections at the bookstore devoted to the proper principles of training, but the basics can be covered quickly. Here's everything you need to know in order to start your efficient, safe workouts.

Form is Everything

"Form" refers to how your body bends and moves in the performance of each lift. The lifts might seem straight forward, but both free-weight and bodyweight movements are quite technical. You might think you know what performing a proper bench press or pull up looks like, but it's surprisingly complicated. At first, when you're using light weights, you can get away with using bad form for a while. Then one day, once you reach a certain weight, you'll get hurt. Not only that, but when you use incorrect form, the lifts won't even build muscle past a certain point. You'll get stuck and have no idea why.

Form doesn't have to be perfect at first but it does need to be pretty good, and done better as you go heavier. Your best option is to hire a coach for a special introductory session of an hour or two, and not just any coach but specifically a strength training coach. Nothing can replace the eye of an experienced trainer when it comes to attaining good form. Due to differences in anatomy, not everyone will look the same when lifting correctly, which is partly why hiring a coach is superior to learning from watching your gym buddy lift.

Can't afford a trainer? Watch online videos, then film yourself with light weights or even a broomstick, comparing your video to theirs. On some websites, you can even post your videos for free "form checks" from your peers or online coaches. Try the forums at Starting Strength (startingstrength.com/resources/forum/), or the subreddit "Form Check" (reddit.com/r/formcheck/). Some excellent YouTube channels I suggest for learning form include Scott Herman Fitness, Athlean-X, Alan Thrall, and the "Art of Manliness" series with Mark Rippetoe.

Each lift has its own things to remember, like foot stance, hand placement, keeping a tight upper back, and squatting below parallel. Lifters will often use "cues" to help remember proper technique as they lift. For example, before a set on the bench press, a lifter might think to himself: "Elbows in," which reminds him to not flare his elbows out, or "Retract scapula," which reminds him to squeeze his shoulder blades together.

Some of these aspects will come naturally, while others will only become second nature after practice. As long as you're doing it mostly right while still on the lighter weights, you'll be okay. Your form will improve with practice. The heavier your lifts get, the closer to perfection your form will need to be. The two main things to always keep in mind from day one are:

1. *If it hurts, stop doing it.* Don't "push through the pain." Change positions or maybe stop doing the lift altogether until you figure out what's wrong. If you still can't do it without pain, try an alternate or variation of the lift.
2. *Don't add weight if it means your form will break down.* Push yourself to keep adding weight but be smart about it. Your ego might require a 250lb bench max, but your body can't cash that check yet.

Mind-Muscle Connection

Closely related to form is the mental connection you have with your muscles. This might sound like hippie talk, but any serious lifter can tell you about it. As you know, all body movement is controlled by the brain. When you lift, your brain releases a chemical neurotransmitter called "acetylcholine" that communicates with your muscles to contract. (McGrath, 2018) We call this communication the mind-muscle connection (MMC).

The better you get at "speaking" to your muscles, the more muscle fibers you'll be able to recruit for each rep, and the better your gains will be. Having a well-developed MMC is necessary for using good form, especially when you're tired and distracted during your workouts. You need to be mentally engaged with each and every rep, and a good MMC will ensure that don't just start going through the motions of lifting. The more you focus on each target muscle group as you lift, the better your lifts will feel, and the more you will experience "the pump."

The pump, by the way, is simply when you can feel your muscles getting engorged with blood. It's the feeling of getting swole, like when you feel your biceps bursting through your shirt sleeve after a set of dumbbell curls. You're most likely to feel the pump when using high-volume sets. What happens is your veins carry blood away from your compressed muscles, blood pools in the muscle, plasma enters the fibers, and those muscle fibers expand and stretch. (Thieme, 2019)

A good MMC will also prevent you from "cheating" on reps. On the bench press, for example, it's easy to lift more weight than you're really capable of lifting (with good form) by simply wrenching and contorting your body. Not only does cheating on reps look silly, it won't make you stronger. Every rep you cheat on essentially doesn't count, but it might get you injured.

To get a better MMC, try these tips courtesy of fitness author Brent McGrath (McGrath, 2018):

- Don't start with a weight that you aren't capable of lifting with good form, i.e. keep your ego out of it. Having more practice at lighter weights will give you time to develop a good MMC.
- Use warm-up sets before every lift to give your mind time to feel each muscle group (before the weight gets heavy).
- Practice your lifts with lighter weight while performing each rep slowly, adding a long pause at the point of the highest muscle contraction (e.g. on bench press, you might pause when the bar is just above your chest, or on squat when you're crouched down just below parallel). This practice can serve as your warm-up sets.
- Flex your muscles between sets to fix your mind on each muscle group. (You might feel like a dork standing there flexing, but it helps.)

Isolation vs. Compound Movements

Compound lifts involve multiple joints and muscle groups at once. For example, the deadlift requires both the hips and knees to bend for a whole-body coordinated effort, which engages the quads, glutes, hams, lats, traps, deltoids, grip strength and the core. (Matthews, Are Compound Exercises Better Than Isolation Exercises?, n.d.)

On the other hand, isolation lifts use only one joint and maybe a few muscle groups at a time. For example, bicep curls, which use only the elbow joint. These are used more for precise body sculpting.

If you want to get big and strong quickly, you need to focus on compound lifts. The workouts are quicker, the whole body gets stronger instead of just a few parts, and you can use more weight and therefore get bigger and stronger. They also signal to your body to produce more natural growth hormones.

Compound lifts can be performed with a barbell, dumbbells, kettlebells, machines, or simply the weight of your own body. The five basic barbell compound lifts are the deadlift, squat, bench press, overhead press, and rows. Compound movements with only bodyweight include lunges, squats, pushups, and pull ups. Each one has different variations and they all work several muscle groups. Adding heavy objects like dumbbells, kettlebells, weighted vests is even better.

A lot of guys only want big arms and chests and don't realize that isolation lifts alone won't get them there. Strength and muscular size aren't the same thing, but they're heavily interconnected. It's a symbiotic relationship where one grows as the other grows, or both stagnate together. If you want to keep getting bigger muscle (on any area on the body), you have to get progressively stronger with heavy, compound lifts.

Sets and Reps

A repetition (or "rep") is one full motion of an exercise. So, one bench press rep means you drop the bar to your chest and push it back up.

A "set" is the number of reps performed in a row without stopping. For example, for squats, 2 sets of 5 reps would mean squatting down and up again 5 times in a row, resting for a moment, then doing it again another 5 times.

A "rep max" (or RM) is the most reps you're able to perform at a certain weight before your body finally can't do any more (known as a "fail"). A 5RM of

100lbs means you can lift 100lbs for five reps before your body gives out during the sixth.

"Intensity" is how heavy the weight is, while "volume" is how much total weight you lift when multiplying reps and sets. High volume training uses light weights but lots of reps, while high intensity training uses heavier weights but with fewer reps and sets. All of these variables combined make up your training "programming."

And note that whenever I refer to using "heavy" weights, I mean whatever weight feels heavy to you, at whatever point in your training you're at. If your one-rep-max on bench press is 150lbs, then a high-intensity lift would be 140lbs for a couple reps, while a high-volume lift would be 80lbs and lots of reps.

How to Choose Which Sets and Reps to Use

Choosing how to train boils down to some simple math (Kamb, 2020):

- To get stronger, denser muscles, do low reps (1 to 5) of heavy weights. Most beginner strength programs use 3 to 5 sets of 5 reps. It's usually the best way to get strong fast.
- To get bigger muscles, do higher reps (6 to 12) of lighter weights.
- To build muscular endurance, do 12 reps or more.

As a beginner, you're better off staying in the 5-rep range at first, and certainly not the 12+. Many strength coaches have found that, for beginners, five reps represent a perfect middle ground between doing too little and too much. The intensity and volume are just high enough to produce more size and strength without over-taxing your system.

This will let you build up a base of raw strength first, so that you can test your strength even further with lower reps later. For now, your strength isn't developed enough for a one-rep-max to have any meaningful effect. Having a solid base of strength will also set you up to handle high reps at heavier weights so you can get huge muscles. Doing very high reps when you're weak won't result in much else than a little cardio.

Intermediates can begin training with higher volume from the get-go. Regardless of you training status or what rep/set combination you choose, pick one and stick with it for a while. Once you stop gaining from it (maybe after a few weeks to months), it's time to find a new rep/set range.

Finally, if you're using bodyweight or dumbbells/kettlebells, you might not have the option to use low reps, at least not for long. This is because you'll soon be strong enough to do several reps with ease. To keep getting stronger, you'll have to make your routine harder, which almost always means lifting weights. The other option is advanced bodyweight exercises which require equipment like rings and weighted vests.

Resting Between Sets

The heavier the weight you're moving, the longer you should rest between sets. With lighter weights you can typically rest as little as 30 to 60 seconds, while for heavier weights it's more like 3 to 5 minutes (and in rare cases up to 10). Lift too early and you might be too fatigued to complete another set, and therefore mistakenly think that that's your new fail number.

Finding Your Starting Weight

The first time you try any movement, you need to start light and work your way up. With dumbbells or kettlebells, start with the lightest one and move to the next until it gets challenging (to the point where you have only a few reps left in the tank by the end of your set).

On a barbell, start with the empty bar itself and only then slowly add 10 pounds at a time. Do this until you reach a weight that feels challenging and that causes your form to start suffering. You'll struggle a little to lift it and the "bar speed" will slow a little. *This is your starting weight.* Continue your first workout with this weight, then move up from here with subsequent workouts. (Rippetoe, Starting Strength: Basic Barbell Training, 2017)

Adding Weight

For lower-body lifts, beginners can add a lot of weight to the barbell with each new workout, typically 10lbs each time for the first few weeks (or even more if you're a bigger guy). When you start failing or really struggling with reps, added weight should drop down to 5 new pounds per workout. The 5-pound jumps will likely last up to several months. Intermediates might need to start with 5-pound jumps.

On upper body lifts like bench press, beginners can start with 5-pound jumps for a few weeks then use "micro plates" of 2.5 pounds or less. (Rodal, 2018) Intermediates might need to start with the micro plates.

Progressing with dumbbells, kettlebells, or weight bodyweight movements is the same principle. You'll slowly lift heavier stuff over time, and the jump in that heaviness will decrease the longer you go.

No matter what, though, every workout should be more challenging than the last, and you should be changing a variable: more weight, more reps, slower reps, etc. Beginner programs will have you adding weight. If you benched 3 sets of 5 reps of 100lbs last workout, now do the same but with 105. When you can no longer add 5lbs per workout, add 2.5, then 2, then 1, and so on. Once you can't add more, and you know you're doing everything else properly—eating, sleeping, and resting enough between sets—then your program is done (and perhaps you're no longer a beginner). It's time to change up your training programming and maybe find a totally different program.

As an intermediate, you'll have to experiment. You might get to a point where adding more weight or reps isn't cutting it. That's when you might experiment with slower reps, faster reps, pause reps, less rest time between sets, pyramid sets, super sets, and so on (whatever it takes to make progress).

Reminder: You will hear veterans talk about their "1 rep max," but as a beginner you shouldn't be testing this yourself. Your nervous system isn't ready for it, and will likely just result in an injury. Just keep making small jumps with low-ish reps. You'll be maxing out soon enough. If you want to know your one-rep-max without actually testing it, do a google search for "one rep max calculator." It will take your current multiple-rep max and extrapolate that into a one-rep-max estimate. For example, if you can squat 150lbs for five reps (i.e. your 5RM), it will tell you your one-rep-max (1RM) is around 170lbs.

How Often and How Long Should I Train?

As a beginner, two to three workouts per week, of a half-hour to one hour per workout, is plenty. Three hours max for the week. You'll need at least one day in between workouts, as recovery usually takes around 48 hours for beginner training sessions. As you move toward intermediate and advanced, you'll recover from workouts faster. Therefore, you can get away with working out more, even every day.

Tracking Your Workouts

Just like your eating, it's important to keep track of your workouts, whether with pen and paper or by using a weight training app. Lots of popular programs offer their own free or paid apps. Write down which lifts you performed, how much weight you used, and number of sets and reps. Make notes of when you fail a rep or something doesn't feel right.

This way you never have to guess how much weight or how many set/reps to use next time. Plus, you'll be able to see your past notes and notice trends with your training. This will help you determine what might be wrong with one particular lift (Rest assured, something *will* go wrong at some point.). Otherwise, without any notes, you'll have no idea what's going on or how to get your training back on track.

Much like your meal prep day, also consider sitting down once a week for a few minutes to write out the workouts you have planned for the upcoming week, or to update your app or spreadsheet.

Warming Up and Stretching

Some people find that it helps to warm up stiff muscles before a workout to prevent injuries. 5 to 15 minutes is usually plenty for strength training. A few common ways to do it include:

- *Cardio*: Jogging, elliptical machine, jump rope, rower machine, etc. It gets the heart rate and body temperature up.

- *Warm-up sets*: This means doing a set of each workout you're about to perform but with a deliberately light weight, no higher than 80% of what you'll be doing during your "real" sets.
- *Stretching*: Warm-ups will usually be enough to prevent most injuries, but stretching can also help, especially for older trainees. However, research shows it might actually be better to stretch after your workout and not before.

Check out Kelly Starrett's YouTube channel for tips on stretching and warming up. Another person worth following is Dr. Caleb Burgess on Instagram, especially if you have mobility issues.

Cardio and Strength Training

While cardio is great for overall health and burning calories, studies show too much of it can actually hinder strength training, especially activities that last more than 30 minutes like long-distance running. This can cut into your recovery and make your muscle gain slower and smaller.

Cardio also has a habit of burning up your hard-earned extra calories. If you're bulking, avoid doing much of it at all, especially if you're a hard-gainer. Your only intense activity during a bulk should be training. If, on the other hand, you gain fat easily, cardio is a good choice.

Beginners who are very weak and unfit should avoid extremely strenuous cardio: sprints, intense rowing, uphill elliptical, etc. Intense cardio can cause "over-training" in these circumstances. For these guys, it's better to use light cardio, even walking for 30 minutes every day or every other day.

If you're cutting or recomping, cardio is excellent. There are some great options for those who want to maintain intense activities during their cut: swimming, cycling, martial arts, and the multi-discipline activity known as "high-intensity interval training." A half hour session a few times per week should be plenty. Again, weaker guys should avoid intense cardio.

Injury vs. Discomfort

A little discomfort from training is normal, including that caused by lactic acid building up in your muscles during workouts (aka "the burn"). All lifters experience a bit of general soreness, aching, stiffness and fatigue after a workout. You might even feel fine after your workout, just to get sore a day or two after. This is called Delayed Onset Muscle Soreness, or "DOMS," and is also an entirely normal experience.

Injuries are different. That's when you experience sharp pain during or immediately after a workout—the kind that makes you wince—or persistent pain, swelling, or inflammation that continues for days or weeks. (Rodal, 2018) (Capritto, 2019) To determine whether a pain is being caused from general soreness or a legitimate injury, keep an eye out for the following signs of injury:

- If the pain is sharp.
- If the pain continues after your warm-up.
- If the pain continues after you've recovered from your workout.
- If only one side of your body hurts but not the other.

Typical lifting injuries occur in the lower back, knees, shoulders, wrists, elbows, and pecs (chest). A common injury for lifters is the "repetitive stress injury." These are nagging pains that aren't debilitating, but will get worse if you ignore them and keep lifting. In these cases, stop doing the particular lift that caused the pain until it resolves. If it still hurts, substitute an alternate variation.

What causes injuries in strength training, and how can you avoid them? Most commonly:

- *Bad form*. It's common for new trainees to get hurt by not knowing how to perform the lifts correctly.
- *Ego*. Don't pick more weight than you can handle just to impress that girl on the other side of the gym. Your form will break down, you'll get hurt, and you'll look dumb.
- *Lack of recovery or rest*. Every workout requires rest in order to recover. If you train without recovering from your last session, you can get hurt.
- *Lack of proper warm up*. Especially for the heavy lifts.

Overtraining and Illness

Working out too much (aka "overtraining") is a very real thing. Your muscles only need a little nudge to get stronger, not a sledgehammer. Don't do more than what your body can recover from, or you might suffer an injury. For beginners, that's only a few hours of training per week. Intermediates can get away with much more. Interestingly, overtraining symptoms tend to be more mental: worsening gym performance, leading to a general malaise and resulting depression, a.k.a. "burnout."

If you feel yourself getting burned out, stop the workouts and focus on resting. The same goes for when you come down with a temporary illness like the flu. If bulking, reduce your calories to maintenance until you're better. Your top priority while sick should be to keep eating enough to not lose any weight and to stay active when possible. You won't lose muscle after only a few days of rest. Just chill until you're better.

Losing Your Gains (and Getting Them Back)

At some point, life will get in the way and your training will have to be put on pause for a while: you'll get really sick for a couple weeks, or you'll have a baby and have no more time to lift, or you'll lose gym access due to a worldwide pandemic. Then, you'll lose muscle and strength. When this happens, don't panic. The fact is, *getting your gains back is a lot easier than when you first got them.*

This is due to "muscle memory," which involves a few things. First, there's your nervous system. As you know, when you first trained, your neural networks got more efficient at moving heavy loads in specific patterns. Even when you detrain for years, your body remembers, and you can regain that strength quickly. In fact, even your DNA remembers. A 2018 study found that, even after detraining for several weeks (and potentially years), your "epigenetic" ability for hypertrophy isn't lost, i.e. if you get swole once and lose it, you can get swole more easily the second time around. (Seaborne et al., 2018)

Finally, there's your muscle cells and their multiple nuclei—called "myonuclei"—which are sort the "control centers" of the cell. During recovery, your individual muscle fibers acquire additional myonuclei from nearby "satellite cells" in order to grow, and BOOM, you get massive pecs and traps. (Tavel, 2018) In a 2010 study of mice, researchers at the University of Oslo discovered that those additional myonuclei tend to stick around after you stop your workouts and your muscles atrophy, potentially for years after (Bruusgaard et al., 2010)

That's all to say this: You've already done the hardest part! Your muscles may have shrunk temporarily, but they remember how to get big, and they can do i fast.

It takes about three to four weeks of not training before muscle begins to break down. (Matthews, n.d.) This is assuming you're not in a calorie deficit and you're still eating enough protein. The first few weeks of not training (aka "detraining") will see a loss of glycogen stores in the muscles (after four weeks, i might be cut in half), a dip in strength, and the loss of some lean mass. Your actual muscle fiber nuclei should stick around for at least three months, if not forever. (Legge, n.d.)

Once you get back to training, you can expect to get back all of you gains in about half the time it took to lose them. So if you lost two months' worth of gains, it should take roughly one month to get them back. If you've detrained for years, that formula doesn't apply. (Nippard, 2020)

However, this doesn't mean you can jump right back into eating and training as when you left off. As you detrained, you lost some strength (both neurological and muscular), you forgot how to lift with good form, and your body isn't capable of recovering from your intense workouts from before. Instead, you'll need to spend a couple weeks (maybe a month) using reduced training volume, intensity, and frequency. Therefore, you'll use fewer sets and reps, with less weight, and work out fewer times per week.

Stay around the 5- to 12-rep range with perhaps only 2-4 sets. No maxing out or going to failure. No lifting six times in a week. Either a Push-Pull-Legs or Upper-Lower routine should be perfect for this. You can easily get all of the necessary volume in just 2-3 workouts per week, 0.5-1 hour apiece. Like normal training, you should still be making your workouts harder each time, but you might do best to avoid adding weight for the first week or two. Instead, make things harder with slow reps, drop sets (not to total failure), pause sets, etc. You should also increase rest between sets since your endurance will be worse.

To avoid muscle soreness, which is common when restarting workouts, use exercises that have less range-of-motion and that feel good. You don't want to over-stretch during lifts (such as lunges) or use a lift where you don't feel a good mind-muscle connection. Cables and machines should be good for this. Continue using heavy compound lifts, but avoid going heavy. Once your strength and

116

form improve after a few weeks, you can get back to lifting hard and heavy like before.

Eating to Get Your Gains Back

As you were forced to stop lifting, you likely let your diet slip. That's okay; it's hard to stay motivated to eat healthy when you don't have any planned lift sessions to put those calories to good use. How you should proceed with your diet as you get back into lifting depends on what happened to your body composition during your training hiatus.

If you continued working out at home during your break—perhaps a bodyweight or dumbbell routine—then you might have kept most if not all of your muscle. If you also ate maintenance calories, then your body composition basically hasn't changed. For the sake of this example, however, I'll just assume you didn't work out hard and that you did lose muscle.

While detraining, hardgainers/ectomorphs will typically reduce calories from a bulk to their natural low-calorie eating habits. Then, they'll lose weight—all muscle loss—while their bodyfat stays the same. Meanwhile, most other guys will lose muscle and gain fat simultaneously, as they detrain. If they ate maintenance calories, they simply lost muscle and gained a higher bodyfat percentage, with no change in weight. If they over-ate during their break, they lost muscle and gained weight (all fat gain).

You already know your dieting choices:

1. *Eat a calorie deficit (i.e. cut).* This is best for anyone who became obese during their hiatus. Build muscle and lose weight, baby.
2. *Eat maintenance calories (i.e. recomp).* This is best for the guys who gained plenty of bodyfat but aren't obese. You can build a little muscle while you lean down.
3. *Eat a calorie surplus (i.e. bulk).* This is best for anyone who doesn't have a significant bodyfat percentage and wants to gain back muscle fast.

Chapter 12 Recap

Using good form with each movement is extremely important, and hiring a coach to learn good form is your best option, although you can use the internet if necessary. You don't have to have perfect form, but it does need to be mostly solid. Two important things to remember about form: don't do a lift if it hurts and don't add weight if your form is no good.

Compound movements are better for getting the whole body big and strong, while isolation lifts are better for gaining size in only certain areas of the body. Compound movements can be performed with weights or simply with your bodyweight.

Every program will have different numbers of sets and reps. Programs focused on getting strong use lower reps (1 to 5) with heavy weights while those focused on getting bigger muscles use higher reps (12+) with relatively lighter weights. You can focus on both equally in the 6 to 12 rep range. The 5 rep range is best for beginners to build a base of strength, after which point you can use higher reps to get bigger. It's difficult (but not impossible) to use the low rep ranges with bodyweight programs. You should rest more between very heavy sets (3 to 5 minutes is typical) and less between lighter sets.

On your first day of training, you have to determine which weights you should start with on each exercise. Do this by slowly adding weight to the empty bar until you struggle to make a rep. After your first day, beginners should add 10lbs to the lower body movements (and then 5lbs per workout). Start with 5-pound jumps on the upper body lifts and then microplates after that. Intermediates will start with smaller jumps. Don't worry about knowing your one rep max for now; it won't help you.

1.5-3 hours per week of training is plenty for a beginner. Intermediates can do more. Track your workouts on paper or on your phone. Record every weight, rep and set, and note when something didn't feel right. This will help you keep your training progress on track.

5 to 15 minutes of a warm up before each workout might help. This means cardio, warm up sets, stretching (consider doing this after your workout instead), or a mix of all of the above. Don't overdo the cardio, especially if you're a novice or hardgainer. Intense cardio is excellent for well-trained guys to burn fat.

Learn the difference between injury and discomfort. Discomfort is normal, whether muscle soreness, stiffness, aches, or fatigue. Injuries are sharp pains, or dull pains that continue after a warm up, after you've recovered from a workout, or that you feel on only one side of the body. Typical lifting injuries occur in the lower back, knees, shoulders, wrists, elbows, and pecs (chest).

118

To avoid injury, avoid using bad form, lifting more than you're capable of, lifting when you aren't fully recovered from a previous workout, and lifting when you haven't adequately warmed up. Also, don't train more than necessary; 2 to 3 hours per week should be plenty. If you get sick, stop working out and focus on maintaining your bodyweight until you're healed.

If you detrain for an extensive period, take two to four weeks to get back into proper shape before continuing your regular training programming. Reduce volume, intensity, and frequency of workouts. With proper diet, expect to get back all of you gains in about half the time it took to lose them. Your diet options include cutting, maintaining, and bulking, and which option is best for you depends on your current detrained body composition.

CHAPTER 13: THE FOUR TYPES OF STRENGTH TRAINING

There are three main types of resistance training (aka strength training), and each has a primary goal with secondary benefits. *Powerlifting* is designed primarily to make you stronger, *Olympic weightlifting* is for developing more explosive power, and *hypertrophy training* (aka bodybuilding) is to grow larger muscles.

When I say strength training, I mean any and all of the above. All three types of training will get you bigger and stronger, but each has a primary benefit. You can try whichever you prefer, and you should consider your goals when choosing. For example, if you're more interested in getting bigger arms than in getting crazy strong, you'll probably prefer a hypertrophy program. Still, you might benefit from a more basic strength program if you're a beginner. Then, after a year at most, you'll be an intermediate, and you can then explore whatever training looks fun.

Like I mentioned in a previous chapter, strength training can be performed with four main methods. Each method will require different equipment and set up. Let's look at them all in detail, as well as the factors into deciding which is best for you.

Barbell Training

This means lifting weight plates that are attached to the ends of a straight metal bar (aka barbell). Common lifts with a barbell include the bench press, deadlift, squats, rows, and overhead press. Barbell training is the best option if you want to get big and strong fast. If you want to do powerlifting or Olympic lifting, you have to train with the barbell.

You only have to learn a few movements to get huge benefits, there are hundreds of lifting variations when you want more variety, it's easy to track your progress, and there's tons of different programs to choose from. Essential equipment includes a squat rack, bench, barbell, and weight set. Or, simply a gym membership.

Dumbbell/Kettlebell Training

This is similar to barbell training, but in this case the weights have their own handles (kettlebells are essentially cannon balls with handles). You can make progress for a lifetime with nothing more than a set of dumbbells or kettlebells. There are tons of programs and all you need is a few pieces of home equipment that you can use in your living room (or, join a gym).

Machine Training

This means lifting weights with a special machine, so that you're actually pushing and pulling a handle that's connected to the weights with tension cables. Common lifts you see with machines but not barbells include leg extensions, cable chest press, and smith machine squats. The downside is, the machines don't test your balance, or strengthen the whole body, as well as free weights do. They're still a good option, but if you prefer to start with machines, I recommend moving on to free weights once you're stronger and more comfortable moving heavy loads.

Bodyweight Training

This is the most basic form of training, since the weight you're lifting is your own body and it's been used for thousands of years. Common exercises include pushups, pull ups, planks, squats, lunges, and so much more. You can put on quite a lot of muscle with just your bodyweight and a few extra pieces of equipment, such as a pull up bar, rings, dip bars, and resistance bands. Programs are easy to follow and the movements relatively easy to learn.

The downside to bodyweight training is you must constantly modify the exercises in order to keep getting stronger. At first, your own weight will be enough to build strength, but eventually you'll need more sophisticated techniques to see any gains. For example, progression might mean going from normal pushups (hands apart) to diamond pushups (hands together), or from regular pull ups to pull ups with added weight.

The possibilities for progressing with bodyweight training are endless. You might progress from running sprints to hill sprint, then hill sprints to weighted hill sprints (with a weighted vest or a sandbag over your shoulder). Hell, you can literally just go to the beach and throw big rocks around; keep using heavier and heavier rocks and you'll get stronger. Still, you should start by finding a program and following a system.

Consider Olympic gymnasts. You know, the guys you see every four years in the Olympics who look extremely lean and jacked. You might be surprised to learn that those guys didn't get their bodies by lifting weights. They primarily gained strength and size with bodyweight movements, especially with the use of rings. Doing "straight-arm" work on rings creates incredible tension on the muscles, and it explains why gymnasts are insanely strong. In fact, these guys are famous for deadlifting double or triple their bodyweight their first time ever touching a barbell. (Shugart 2004)

Make no mistake, you can get absolutely jacked with just a bodyweight routine. Former NFL great Hershel Walker grew up as a short and chubby kid, with no athletic ability and no extra money for gym equipment. In sixth grade, he began an intense daily routine of mostly pushups, pull ups, sit ups, and hill sprints. By high school, Walker was a beast, and he went on to be one of the greatest pro football players of all time. (McKay B. M., 2020) It goes to show, you don't need a bunch of fancy equipment to get ripped.

Find What Works for You

As a beginner, you should find a basic program and see it through for at least a few months. Once it's complete, the world is your oyster, and your options for exercise selection will be endless. Don't want to be limited to one type of training? Do a mix of all of them. Some programs have a lot of exercise variety so you can try what interests you.

Want to set up a home gym but can't afford home equipment new from the store? Keep your eye out at Craigslist, social media marketplaces, thrift stores, and local auctions. Don't want to shell out extra for that personal trainer at the gym? Watch YouTube videos. Are you dealing with mobility issues? Do more comfortable bodyweight exercises or machines instead of barbells.

What works for your buddy might not work for you, and a program that a celebrity swears will get you huge might do you little good. Some movements will work better for you than for others. Same with set/rep schemes. Over time, you'll figure out what does and doesn't work. It's important to give a new program time and to be sure you're following it correctly, but if it just isn't working for you, move on.

Coach Dan John puts it this way: "I am giving you the secret of my four decades of sports performance: Once you know what works for you, it is always going to work for you to some degree. And, on the contrary, if something doesn't...my friend, run screaming from it." (John, Mass Made Simple: A Six-Week Journey into Bulking, 2020)

Do Something You Enjoy

"If you think of exercise as a 60-minute commitment 3 times a week at the gym, you're missing the point completely. If you think that going on a diet has something to do with nutrition, you don't see the forest through the trees. It is a lifestyle. I know it sounds cliché, but you have to find things you love to do."
—Brett Hoebel, Celebrity Trainer

It's important to choose a workout routine that you can stick to for at least a few months. If you're a beginner, your "newbie gain" phase won't last forever, so it's important to train hard while it lasts. Whether bulking, cutting, or recomping, you want to be sure your calories are going to good use. If you can't stand the first program you choose, find another one quickly. We're not all wired the same. Some people do the same three exercises over and over and over, and they love it. Others need more variety.

Not every workout will be "fun," but you should at least be motivated enough to do it. It's a common myth that fitness junkies "love to work out."

Sometimes, sure, but not always. Muhammad Ali famously said that he hated every minute of training. (Don't worry though, your training probably won't be nearly as intense as his was.) Just keep with it and there's a good chance you'll end up a fitness junkie yourself.

Consistency, Not Perfection

You don't need to do this whole thing perfectly. Don't fail to get started because you're unsure what's the perfect rep range for you, or which specific lifts will get you bigger arms, or which adjustable dumbbell has the best ergonomics. These are minor details. Just start a good, proven program and be consistent. In other words, "Just show up."

Consistency Is key. Miss a workout because something came up? Don't beat yourself up; just work out tomorrow. Failed a rep? That's fine, you'll get it next time. Couldn't sleep last night and now you have no energy to lift? No big deal, it's a minor hiccup. Hate your new workout routine? Don't skip it, just start a new one.

If you stick with it, the gains will add up, and you'll see the difference in the mirror soon enough. It's like dropping coins in a piggybank. It doesn't seem like much each time, but after a few months you can buy yourself something spiffy.

On the other hand, it's pointless to train inconsistently, because you'll make virtually no progress. You need to get in a certain amount of volume week-to-week, every week. If you skip a week and then try to sneak in all the necessary work in one day, that's just three steps back, one step forward. The only option is to train regularly—at least 2 to 3 times per week—to spread the volume out.

Training, in and of itself, is pretty easy. Anyone can do it for a day. The hard part is being consistent. It's forcing yourself to work out when you're tired or "too busy." It's choosing to stick with a planned workout instead of meeting your friends for happy hour. Being consistent is what will separate you from most other guys at the gym.

Chapter 13 Recap

Barbell training means lifting weights with a barbell and performing lifts like bench press, squat, and deadlift. It's the best option for getting big and strong quickly. Dumbbell and kettlebell training require less equipment and you can still get huge gains. Machine training (such as with cable machines) is a good and safe way to gain muscle.

Bodyweight training is the simplest and cheapest option. Compound movements like squats, pushups, and pull ups are your go to. Add in weighted vests and other special equipment to continue gaining size and strength.

Do whatever type of training that works best for you, because what works for one person won't work best for everyone. If you aren't getting decent gains or your body doesn't feel comfortable doing one type of training, find another one.

Do whatever keeps you motivated. Not every workout will be fun, but you should find something you're willing to keep doing for months at a time. Also, don't worry about finding the perfect program; just pick one and get started. Train consistently and the gains will add up; you can only expect results if you train often, at least 2 to 3 times per week.

CHAPTER 14: CHOOSING A PROGRAM AND A GYM

There are literally thousands of workout programs to choose from, but I'll help you narrow it down. Whatever you choose, it doesn't have to be perfect. It just needs these few key things:

1. *Is it simple?* The more complicated a program is, the harder it is to know what is and isn't working. Remember the old mantra, "Keep It Simple, Stupid." The best recipe (for beginners especially) is to start with a very basic program, just a handful of movements (four or five is plenty, but more is okay), and an easy-to-remember structure of reps/sets. Once you get the hang of it, then you can add other stuff (e.g. isolation lifts and accessory work).

2. *Does it include full-body compound movements?* It should. You don't have to do super heavy squats and deadlifts, but you should at least do full-body movements that are similar to them. Most of the big lifts can be substituted with weighted bodyweight movements. For example, substitute kettlebell goblet squats for barbell squats, or weighted pullups for rows. Again, to get as big and strong as possible, barbell training is your best option. Isolation lifts are fine too, but they aren't necessary. In fact, for a beginner, they might not even help until you've built significant strength.

3. *Is it designed for your type?* Some programs are meant just for beginners, while others are for intermediate or advanced trainees. Some are just for women, some for just men. Some are designed for tall, skinny guys. Others for just young, athletic guys. And so on. Don't pick a program that's designed for someone else.

4. *Have other people like you had success with it?* If so, it'll probably work for you too. Stick to programs that are well-known; this way, you know it's worked for thousands. Avoid new, trendy workouts.

5. *Does it allow for long-term progress?* You want a program that provides progressive overload for more muscle and strength with each new workout, not just for weeks but for at least a few months. Avoid trendy "listicle" programs like the "Get Python Arms in 30 Days" nonsense you see advertised online.

6. *Will it get you to your goal?* If you want to get really strong, for example, don't choose a program with lots of isolation lifts or really light weights. If you're trying to gain as much mass as possible and quickly, you'll have to use heavy weights with compound lifts.

7. *Can you realistically stick to it?* Don't pick a program that requires working out 6 days a week, for example, if you hate working out. Likewise, don't pick a program with only a few exercises if you need more variety in your workouts.

Remember to find something you enjoy. After being an athlete for over four decades, Dan John realized that the way we are "wired to work" has a major impact on our training. He noted that some people can stick with a program for years, while most others tend to quit any program they try after the first few weeks. (John, Mass Made Simple: A Six-Week Journey into Bulking, 2020)

Starting Strength and Other Beginner Barbell Programs

If you're a beginner and you want to lift with barbells, there are several programs that are extremely popular and guaranteed to work for you. Each of these programs should allow for a few months of linear progression. Once you start stalling on lifts or you can't recover from your workouts, it will be time to move on to an "advanced beginner" or intermediate program.

The first is called "Starting Strength." Possibly the most popular beginner barbell program of all time, it's low volume and heavy weight. It's simple to follow and there's only five lifts to learn. You'll have three workouts per week of 45 to 60 minutes apiece. It's best for young athletes, but it's good for all ages, anyone who wants to get strong fast. The program shouldn't last more than a few months (perhaps only three). You can learn the program via the book *Starting Strength: Basic Barbell Training* by program creator Mark Rippetoe, perhaps *the* definitive book about weight lifting. You can also learn the basics at their website (startingstrength.com/about), ask questions to coaches, get free form checks, and

127

read diet and lifting advice from pros. They also offer an app and paid online coaching. The downside is the program focuses more on lower body than some guys prefer, and it focuses more on raw strength than muscular size.

"Strong Lifts 5x5" is very similar to Starting Strength. It's mostly low-volume but with more emphasis on upper body. "5x5" simply means you will do five sets of five reps on each lift (on the days you use those lifts). Like Starting Strength, this program can last months. It's reputable, simple to follow, and has a handy app, although your workouts will be a little longer (90 minutes). Thousands have had success with this program. Learn the basics at (stronglifts.com/5x5/).

"GreySkull LP" is a three day per week routine for beginners. It was designed to be similar to Starting Strength and Strong Lifts but with more volume.

"Ice Cream Fitness 5x5" requires three workouts per week, 90 minutes per workout, and it should last around 12 weeks. It offers more lifts and exercise variety than the aforementioned programs.

"Westside for Skinny Bastards (WS4SB)" is similar to Starting Strength in that it's perfect for skinny hardgainers to get big and strong fast. It's three long workouts per week with tons of exercise variety. You can actually choose which lifts you prefer and which ones "feel" right for you. You'll have to spend considerable time learning the movements.

Programs for Tall Guys

Any basic barbell program will help a beginner add strength and size for a while, regardless of his height. There's nothing wrong with tall beginners using a program like the ones described above. However, as the weights get heavier and heavier, and as you transition to intermediate after a few months to a year, tall guys will start running into unique problems.

Moving heavy weight around can be awkward for taller guys, unless you have a big "Strongman"-type frame, which you probably don't. You probably have a narrow skeletal frame and long, thin arm and leg bones (especially the humerus and femur). Think of these long limbs as your "levers." Having longer levers means you have to move further and do more work to squat, for example, compared to someone shorter.

According to veteran trainer Alexander Cortes, heavy movements can be stressful on tall people's joints. You have a harder time building muscle, and you can't achieve as much pure strength. (Cortes, Tall Man Training: The Strategies and Principles for Taller Men in Lifting, 2020) I've seen this warning repeated by numerous trainers. The warning is basically that tall guys shouldn't try elite powerlifting, and they shouldn't expect normal programs to give them huge muscles like with shorter-limbed guys.

There are a number of ways to combat this. One is to *use more reps*. A "5-Rep" program like Starting Strength will certainly get you stronger and bigger, but eventually you'll want to find something with more volume. If you want huge arms, you'll need more reps. According to coach Dan John, guys with long limbs and on the taller side need more reps and more time with a load in their hand to get bigger. (John, Mass Made Simple: A Six-Week Journey into Bulking, 2020) The taller you are and the heavier you go with any low-rep lift, the more issues you'll likely run into. For example, you might have no issue squatting 200lbs, but as you approach 300 or 400, it's likely you'll start experiencing some issues (despite using good form). Don't sacrifice your healthy knees and shoulders for more gains.

Another way to avoid tall-guy problems is to *use more variety* in your training and don't rely solely on the big lifts like bench, deadlift, and squat. Things like dumbbells, cables, machines, and weighted bodyweight movements will be an excellent way to gain muscular size. If a certain lift feels awkward or you can't feel your muscles engaging properly, then that lift probably isn't for you. Try a variation of it—like incline bench instead of regular, or dumbbell rows instead of barbell—or drop the lift altogether.

Search for More Lifting Options

The internet is full of free and paid workout routines, at reliable fitness websites like Bodybuilding.com, MuscleAndFitness.com, NerdFitness.com, and many more. Just be sure the program is meant for you.

I suggest reading "The 12 Best Science-Based Strength Training Programs for Gaining Muscle and Strength" over at LegionAthletics.com. The author breaks down 12 programs, some of which I've already mentioned, including many for beginners.

You can also do specific internet searches. Want to do a split routine such as upper-lower or push-pull-legs? Maybe you prefer a dumbbell-only or kettlebell-only routine? Maybe you'd like a mix of some lifting and some exercises you can do outdoors? Prefer to do several short workouts per week vs. a couple long workouts? Perhaps you want a program designed specifically for your body type (e.g. training for tall men)? Search specifically for those.

Want to avoid certain types of lifts? Search for programs that exclude the ones you know you don't like. This will be especially useful for intermediates who already have a decent idea of what types of movements they prefer. For example, Jason Helmes of AnyManFitness.com has a program designed specifically to get jacked without having to do heavy squats and deadlifts. This isn't to say you should skip every lift you don't like, but you do have options. Jason is one of hundreds of reputable trainers that offer online coaching as well.

By the way, "Never skip leg day" is a popular saying for good reason. You don't have to lift legs every workout, but you shouldn't totally neglect them. This is for a few reasons: You'll end up looking silly with giant arms and little chicken legs; you'll lack any serious athletic ability without lower body strength; a lack of muscular balance will make you more prone to injury; the big lower body lifts create the most muscle, which creates a more anabolic environment to get upper body gains; finally, missing out on these lower body muscle gains means missing out on a faster metabolism for burning fat in the future.

Bodyweight Routines

The subreddit /r/bodyweightfitness is a good forum for learning and asking questions about bodyweight routines. Their "Recommended Routine" and "Training Guide" are an excellent choice for getting started.

This beginners guide at nerdfitness.com is also good choice for learning the basics, especially if you start very weak: The Beginner Bodyweight Workout. Although, this programming won't last long, and you'll soon need to find a more advanced program.

Onnit.com offers a great choice for progressing all the way from beginner to advanced, and it includes video instructions: Basic to Beast Complete Bodyweight Program.

CrossFit

Although CrossFit is hugely popular right now, it unfortunately won't help you build lots of muscle long term, especially if you're trying to gain weight. CrossFit focuses more on burning calories and getting generally more fit. You know those CrossFit athletes you see on Instagram looking extremely jacked and lean? They didn't get that way using CrossFit; they got it via conventional strength training. Same for anything else that's high intensity for long durations, such as MMA, P90X, Orange Theory, and others. These programs are great for maintaining muscle and burning calories to stay lean, but building more muscle, not so much.

After the Beginner Phase

As you know, after training consistently for a few months to a year, you'll likely go from a beginner to an intermediate trainee. This is when you'll need a new program if you want to keep achieving gains, and there's tons of programs to choose from.

For barbell training that focuses on pure strength, go with a low-volume program. Here's a few famous intermediate powerlifting routines (all are free online):

- Jim Wendler's 5/3/1
- The Texas Method
- Madcow 5x5
- TSA Program
- Candito 6-Week Program
- Calgary Barbell 8- & 16-Week Program
- Greg Nuckols Intermediate Program

I'm including this article from liftvault.com which explains most the above programs. It also includes free downloads of Excel templates for each program which you can print at home (https://liftvault.com/programs/powerlifting/top-5-intermediate-powerlifting-programs/).

If instead of building pure strength, you want your intermediate program to focus more on building bigger muscles, use a bodybuilding routine (aka hypertrophy training). I'm including a second article from liftvault.com, this one describing ten of the best bodybuilding routines out there. Some are for beginners, while most are for either intermediate or advanced trainees (or both). You'll also be able to download free spreadsheets to print and follow (https://liftvault.com/programs/bodybuilding/)

Powerlifting and bodybuilding aren't your only options, either. There's still Olympic lifting, dumbbell routines, kettlebell routines, bodyweight programs, and more, all ranging from intermediate to advanced.

If you want to take a deep-dive into the world of kettlebell training, Pavel Tsatsouline is good pro to learn from, but there are books and Youtube videos with hundreds of reputable pros. Or, check out sites like Onnit.com for free routines.

Joining A Gym

Joining a gym can be intimidating if you're a beginner. You might be self-conscious about working out next to people who are more fit and experienced. Plus, you might not even know how to navigate the space.

But to ease your fears quickly, let me point out that not even gym veterans know how every single machine there works. Most gym staffs are excited to have you there, and will show you around and explain the equipment during your first visit. They'll also break down all the additional services you can get for more pay, from personal trainers to massages, sports medicine and more.

If you're feeling insecure about your body or fitness level, or the fact that you don't know how to perform the lifts yet...I get it. Most of the other gym-goers get it too, and they will respect the hell out of you just for showing up and putting in the effort. They started from zero just like you're doing. Try not to concern yourself with the opinions of the few people there who are judgmental. Instead, make friends with the much larger group of people who are cheering you on.

Your mission for your first workout is to learn the layout and rules of that gym, and to figure out your starting weight for the various exercises that your program requires for that day. Your first full workout shouldn't be rushed or overly taxing, so take your time and don't be afraid to ask lots of questions to the staff. That's why you're paying them to be there, after all. Bring a bag, water bottle, your lift journal or phone, a towel to wipe off both yourself and the equipment, and of course shower supplies and a change of clothes if you're going to bathe there afterwards.

Squat shoes help with squats but aren't absolutely necessary. Flat footed shoes are best for deadlifts. Otherwise, wear what's comfortable, but avoid running shoes or any other shoe that has a lot of bounce. You want your feet to be firmly planted to the ground when you lift, not bouncing every time you shift your weight. Wear tops and bottoms that allow your body to stretch.

Be considerate. Try to get in and out in a reasonable time period, and don't hog a machine while you scroll on your phone (unless you're just resting between sets). Put weights back when you're done. Wipe your sweat off the equipment. If someone asks you to "spot" them, tell them you haven't done it before, or ask how to best help (but don't feel obligated).

Chapter 14 Recap

Your training program should be all of these things: simple, includes compound movements, designed for your body type and level of training, has a successful track record, allows for long-term progress, will get you to your goals, and you can realistically stick to it.

"Starting Strength" and programs like it are excellent choices for beginners that want to get big and strong fast. They require three workouts per week, around 60-90 minutes apiece, and there are tons of online resources to learn all about the programs.

Tall guys need to train differently than others due to your long limbs. You can still get strong with the aforementioned programs, but eventually you need to get in more volume (i.e. use more reps and sets with lighter weights) and more variety of exercises than the big barbell lifts.

To find other programs that better suit you, search the internet for specifically what you want. It can be based on your body type, which lifts you prefer to perform, which equipment you'd rather use, and which type of weekly routine you would prefer. CrossFit and other similar high-cardio mixed programs won't help you get much bigger. After your first few months to year of consistent training, you'll go from being a beginner to an intermediate. This means you'll have to find a new program.

Joining a gym can be intimidating but the gym staff and fellow lifters will make it much easier. Gym staff will show you the gym layout and how all the equipment works, and will offer you paid services like personal training. Everyone at that gym started from zero like you are doing now, and the vast majority of them will be kind and supportive. For your first workout, focus on learning the layout and rules of the gym, and figure out your starting weights on each exercise.

Necessary gym equipment: a bag, water bottle, journal or phone, towel, shower supplies (if needed), squat shoes (if preferred), and clothes that stretch adequately. Remember to be considerate of other gym members by not hogging equipment, putting weights up, wiping down the equipment after, and assisting other members that need help with a spot.

CHAPTER 15: WHEN THE GOING GETS TOUGH

Every fitness book seems to have a section on motivation, and they're almost always cheesy. "Believe in yourself" might be good and all, but I can't say it ever encouraged me to slam down a protein shake with zero appetite. I don't know about you, my friend, but mantras just don't pump me up. Platitudes like "live every day to the fullest" have as much impact on me as when someone tells me they "love to laugh."

On the other hand, a good quote from someone with real life experience is helpful. Henry Ford is one such person. The famous industrialist had this to say about believing in yourself: "Whether you think you can, or you think you can't, you're right." Thomas Jefferson put it this way: "Nothing can stop the man with the right mental attitude from achieving his goal; nothing on earth can help the man with the wrong mental attitude."

Your new diet and training *will* lead to some aggravation at the very least. Some days you'll want to give up, and that's normal. I've been there many times these past few years. Here's a few things for you to keep in mind.

Remember Why You're Doing This

"Twenty years from now, you will be more disappointed by the things you didn't do than by the ones you did do. So throw off the bowlines. Sail away from the safe harbor. Catch the trade winds in your sail. Explore. Dream. Discover."

—Mark Twain

In his book *Never Let Go*, coach Dan John explains what he learned about motivating athletes after four decades of experience. He said that you shouldn't focus on the pleasure of achieving your goal. Instead, *focus on the pain of not achieving your goal.* (John, 2009) Don't think, "I'll look good if I get fit and that'll be awesome." Eating churros on the couch and watching cooking shows all day is awesome too. Believing that you'll look good in a few months isn't enough to motivate most people when their diet and workouts get hard. In other words, you can't just *want* something badly enough; you have to *need* it.

Instead, you might think to yourself, "I need to be healthier because degenerative disease runs in my family," or "I can't let my childhood crush see me like this at the class reunion," or "I need to be healthy enough down the road to play with my grandkids." This is the stuff that really drives us.

In another book, *Mass Made Simple*, John mentions a "diet" once devised by a famous performance consultant called the "Alpo Diet." Here's how it worked. You tell all your friends that you're going to lose 10 pounds in a month, and if you don't lose it all by then, they have permission to force you to eat a can of Alpo dog food in front of them. For the next month, you'll avoid brownies and ice cream like the plague.

His point was this: "Most people would rather avoid pain than embrace joy or pleasure… When you need some encouragement, crack open the can and sniff some Alpo and, for whatever reason, you'll tend to stick to the plan!" (John, Mass Made Simple: A Six-Week Journey into Bulking, 2020)

Obviously, don't actually eat dog food. (At least, don't let your friends watch.) My version of dog food was imagining a lifetime of being small and never having the life I really wanted. The most painful part was imagining myself as a frail older man full of regret, knowing I could have done something about it. I *needed* to get big.

What's your dog food?

136

It Gets Easier

It might be overwhelming at first to start eating new foods and bigger meals, making new recipes, learning a new training program, having a new schedule, etc. But you will adjust. Day one will be much harder than day 50. These things will slowly become second nature to you, and your healthy choices will soon become habits. (Read James Clear's *Atomic Habits* if you want to understand more of the science behind how this works.)

Pretty soon you'll start looking forward to your workouts, because now you're seeing results and the progress is exciting. The training principles you read about will start to make more sense as you live them out. You'll also have more natural energy to work out. Your cravings for sugar will go down so much that now ignoring that box of apple fritters in the break room feels like a no-brainer. You'll start to feel pretty good about the way you're spending your time, instead of laying on your couch for eight straight hours playing vidya games. Everything will start to feel easier, even mundane physical tasks like picking up an Amazon package off the ground.

It gets *even easier* in the long-term. As you know, staying in shape is a lot easier than getting in shape in the first place. Still, you might be picturing getting jacked and then having to lift weights for the rest of your life or you'll shrink back down to your old scrawny self. In reality, you just have to stay active to stay fit. Ever heard of "old man strength?" It's when you see an older gentleman who doesn't work out and yet he's strong as an ox. There's a good chance he built up a lot of size and strength in his teens and twenties playing football or working on the family farm. Now, to maintain his fitness, all he does is hike, chop wood, and eat meat and vegetables. It really is that easy.

You'll Get Tougher

Being big and strong is not the same as being "tough." Plenty of muscle-bound fitness enthusiasts are total babies when it comes to experiencing basic hardships like harsh weather and general stress. You know, the guys who will complain about a paper cut? This was me, until I got a job that forced me to do manual labor in 100-degree heat, hike miles in heavy snowfall, and trek through rattlesnake-infested fields. (I actually learned to love it.)

The thing about toughness is, it's a skill that can be trained. To get tougher, you have to do things that are uncomfortable. Of course, we live in relatively comfortable times now. When our not-too-distant ancestors traveled across country, it was on rickety wagons, often passing through hostile areas, with a high risk of disease and malnutrition, and the trips could last months. Now, we casually drive a few hours in our air-conditioned SUVs while listening to a murder-mystery podcast and sipping hot coffee from an insulated cup. The worst thing that might happen is you burn your lip.

These days, you have to seek out hardship (aka voluntary hardship). For some people, this might mean taking cold showers, fasting, or exercising in a hot garage. Bulking and strength training are no different. You'll be dealing with an entirely new type of stress that you might be unaccustomed to, and you'll toughen up quick.

Not just the physical aspects either (hand callouses, body soreness, etc.). You'll toughen up mentally too: You'll learn to ignore other people's opinions of you when you're a newbie struggling to lift light weights; You'll get better at facing frustrating problems, like when you stall on a lift and have to figure out a solution; You'll learn to persevere through intense workouts when you'd rather go home and rest. All of these things will make you more resilient in adversity.

Trust the Process

Don't expect change overnight. It takes time, and you won't see visible results in the mirror on a day-to-day basis. Take progress pics every couple of weeks and then you'll see the slow change. You won't enjoy taking these photos at first, but you'll be glad afterwards that you did it. Worst case scenario, after a few months of bulking and lifting, it might even seem like you've only added a small layer of fat rather than bulging muscles. Don't worry, if your strength has improved significantly, then the muscle is there.

On a personal note, my coworkers were confounded by my dieting habits: drinking milk half-a-gallon at a time, refusing to eat the office donuts, and eating basically the same thing every day. Instead of being embarrassed by the whole thing, I embraced the fact that I was accomplishing something that couldn't be seen. Soon enough, it became obvious by my progress why I was doing it.

Also, rest assured, these odd eating habits won't last forever. Just a few months should be enough to add serious pounds. You might feel ridiculous bringing your own healthy meals to work (instead of eating fast food with your coworkers), snacking at your desk as people stare, and drinking milk like a toddler. You'll be back to your regularly scheduled programming of normal meals in no time.

It's More About the Journey Than the Destination

It sounds cliché, mostly because it is, but nonetheless it's true. A new body will be awesome, but your new confidence from this experience will be the real game changer. A month or two into bulking seriously, you'll see exactly what I mean.

Life experience is what builds confidence. You start by making decisions and taking action, which requires some courage. When you act, you get results, and those results build confidence. "Fake it 'til you make it" might work for a while, but it's not the real thing. Famous public orator William Jennings Bryan put it like this: "The way to develop self-confidence is to do the thing you fear and get a record of successful experiences behind you."

There's plenty of things to fear when it comes to bulking: letting others see you fail, getting hurt from lifting heavy weights, gaining fat when you know losing fat is difficult, and so on. Taking action in the face of these fears will do more for you than reading a million motivational quotes.

You're Not the First Person to Do This

Thousands upon thousands of men have bulked up successfully. We've all been where you are right now. We've all experienced the overwhelming feeling of having to adopt a whole new lifestyle, the workouts where we felt weak, the times in the gym when we felt incapable of getting over a plateau, the big meals where we didn't think we could eat another bite, and the times we took our pictures and weren't sure we had changed at all.

Your bulking program will have some setbacks: You'll miss a rep in your workout and have to figure out why; You'll feel like you ate a ton of food one day and then realize you're still short a few hundred calories; You'll wake up on morning and realize you actually lost a little weight.

These things will happen and that's to be expected. It doesn't mean you'r failing; when you keep going, it means you're someone who doesn't give u easily. We've all wanted to give up at some point. Former MLB coach Michae Boyle explained it best when he said, "Most people give up right before the bi break comes — don't let that person be you."

Death by A Thousand Excuses

There will always be an excuse to not work out, or not eat a healthy mea "I'm busy today." "I'm tired." "I feel too bloated to eat more." All reasonabl enough. My advice: *ignore them.*

Make time for your workout even if it means waking up earlier. Drink tha protein shake like it's your second job. You can quit your day job at any time right? Why don't you? It's because your job is important, people are counting o you, and your reputation and livelihood are on the line. Even more, you want t keep your paychecks coming. Sticking with your scheduled workouts anc healthy meals is the same way. The "wants" just have to outweigh the "don' wants."

Of course, sometimes you'll have legitimate reasons to skip a workout or t eat Wendy's instead of a healthier option. That's fine; sometimes life gets in the way. However, if you're like me, your excuses will usually be just that, excuses As Arnold Schwarzenegger said, "You can have results or excuses, but not both." He would know. A more accurate (and nerdier) way of putting it: results anc excuses have an inverse relationship; the more excuses you succumb to, the les results you'll get.

Use the Drive That's Already in You

All right, despite what I said earlier, this part might get kind of cheesy. But it' the truth.

Think back to a time in your life when you were faced with something scar *and you did it anyway.* Maybe it's when you talked to your crush, had that jot

140

interview or that home improvement project where you felt way over your head, or when you were scared to jump your bike but didn't want your friends to see you wuss out.

What did all those events have in common? You wanted something, you were afraid to do it because of what might happen, but you did it anyway. You may not have ultimately succeeded, but you at least had the guts to try it.

Showing courage doesn't mean you stop feeling fear or anxiety; it means you're willing to act in spite of those feelings. That kettlebell or that thousand-calorie shake in front of you is just another boogeyman hiding in the closet, and you need to face it. Once again, the Terminator put it best when he said, "When you go through hardships and decide not to surrender, that is strength."

Chapter 15 Recap

To deal with the hard times of bulking: Remember what is driving you to make this change, and remember why you *need* this (i.e. your "dog food"). Know that it will get easier over time; the diet and workouts will become second nature. You'll also get even tougher. Think long term, trust the process, and remember that this will only last a few months before you can eat more normally again. Also, enjoy that new confidence you feel; it's very real and well earned.

Remember that thousands upon thousands of other guys have been through exactly what you're about to embark on. We all have lots of excuses to not diet and train as we're supposed to, and while some of these excuses are perfectly valid, most of them are best to ignore. Finally, don't let a little fear stop you; you've faced it a thousand times before.

CHAPTER 16: FAQ AND YOUR TO-DO LIST

Frequently Asked Questions

"Do I still have to overeat on days that I don't work out?" Yup. Every day, you need to overeat when you're bulking. It's on your rest days that you do most of your recovery, and that's when you need the extra calories the most. Don't freak out that you're stuffing your face without working out on the same day. It's all part of the plan.

"Can I do intermittent fasting?" You technically can but realistically shouldn't. It will make bulking nearly impossible. Save it for cutting and recomping.

"Does soreness mean I'm getting stronger?" Maybe. A lack of soreness probably means you're not building muscle, but being sore doesn't prove you are.

"What if I don't know enough to know what I'm doing?" It's normal to feel overwhelmed by so much information, but you do know enough to get started. When you have questions, use your trainer and the internet (and revisit this book).

"What if my training program stops working?" See Mark Rippetoe's free online article "The First 3 Questions" (startingstrength.com/article/the_first_three_questions). It's a short, easy read.

142

Unless you've been following the program successfully for several months (in which case, it's simply run its course and time to find a new program), most likely you're not following your program correctly. The main three ways you can sabotage your program: You're not resting enough between sets; You're adding too much weight each workout; You're not recovering (i.e. not eating enough, not eating the right stuff, or not sleeping enough). (Rippetoe, The First Three Questions, 2015)

"Will I have to bulk forever to maintain my new weight?" No, you can technically stay the same weight via transitioning to a recomp. If you're doing a bulk and suddenly drop calories significantly, you'll lose weight. If you do continue bulking, it won't require as large a surplus over time.

"Can I quit working out and eating healthy after I reach my body goals?" You can work out less often or less intensely, but you can't just stop and expect to keep the body you've earned. Fortunately, you don't have to train nearly as hard to maintain muscle as you did to build it. Your diet, though, will still require high protein and mostly whole foods to stay lean and ripped. I will say this: once you've gotten lean and muscular, your body will allow a lot more "cheating" without getting fat. Partly because your nutrition partitioning will have improved so significantly that your body will put a slice of pizza to much better use now than it would have before you were fit (i.e. the protein in that pizza is more likely to go toward muscle-building that fat-storage).

"What if I don't eat enough calories one day?" If you miss your calorie target one day, you can usually make up for it later. For example, if your bulk calls for 3,000 kcal per day and you only eat 2,800 on Monday, then eat 3,200 on Tuesday and it will even out. Generally, as long as you eat enough surplus between workouts, and you're not having extreme swings in intake (e.g. eating zero one day and 6,000 the next), you're good.

"Can I gain or lose weight in specific body areas?" Unfortunately, no. At least, not in the sense that dieting alone can do it, despite the ads that tell you otherwise. Weight gain or loss is mostly distributed evenly through the whole body. It depends on your genetics too. Some bodies are predisposed to add weight to one area first, like the midsection, and that's also where you lose it last. As you body

composition improves via training, your weight will distribute in more attractive ways.

"Is it true that when you gain fat you grow new fat cells that never go away?" This is true, but your new fat cells will shrink when you do a cut. (Preiato, 2020) It's also true that because of your new fat cells, you might gain fat more easily in the future. Although, adding more muscle mass (which bolsters your metabolism) simultaneously should offset this negative side effect. Bulking intelligently to minimize fat gain will also help prevent the issue of future fat gain.

"What if I'd rather work out at home?" There's plenty of guides online on how to build a home gym safely and cheaply.

"Will I have to buy a whole new wardrobe?" You'll probably need new pants with a larger waist size (at least for the first few months of bulking), but that should be the only new purchase necessary. Your shirts will likely start to fit better.

"Is it true that bulkers have bad acne break outs?" It's true that some bulkers report their acne getting worse. Based on my research, it seems to be mostly due to eating unhealthily (especially processed junk food). However, some bulkers have reported dairy as the culprit, especially milk. If you consume a lot of dairy and experience a worsening of your acne, that could be the cause.

"What if I still can't gain weight after reading this book?" You might benefit from a one-on-one approach, and you should consider hiring a coach or nutritionist. Also, remember the articles I recommend under "Homework for Hardgainers."

"Why is there so much conflicting info on bulking?" There's a number of reasons for this:

- *Dishonesty.* Snake oil peddlers promise unrealistic gains. Remember, if it sounds too good to be true, it almost certainly is.
- *Lack of research.* Most studies regarding weight are focused on losing it rather than gaining it. Thankfully there's enough research to still know what we're doing, but it's a major factor into why you see so many different numbers floating around.

- *Anecdotal stories.* Someone hears over beers about a friend of a friend who once gained 40lbs of muscle in a year, and assumes it's a true story that happened exactly the way they heard it. Unfortunately, even some pros in the fitness world promote these stories.
- *Steroids.* Some bodybuilders (and notoriously a lot of celebrities) take drugs to get quick muscle gains with minimal fat gains, but fail to tell the public that's how they got it.

"Why isn't the advice in this book more popular and why doesn't everyone do it?" Because it's hard. Fad diets and 30-day training programs are lying to you. The real transformation happens over many months and years and with a ton of consistent effort. It takes hard work that most people aren't willing to do. This is true for anything in diet and fitness. Take the "Tabata" workout, for example, which can take less than five minutes and arguably burns more fat than an hour of jogging. So, why doesn't everyone use Tabata instead of jogging? Because Tabata is a whole lot harder.

Your To-Do List

As we wrap up, I want to give you a final reminder of everything you need to accomplish in order to begin your entire bulking program. In no particular order:

1. Write out your goals, your reasons for bulking, and realistically what you can put into it.
2. Calculate your maintenance calories, Body Mass Index, and bodyfat percentage; approximate your body type.
3. Choose your desired caloric surplus and macro percentages based on your unique factors: age, BMI, bodyfat percentage, body type, genetic potential, and goals.
4. Make a grocery list and meal plans for the first week or two. Consider downloading a grocery list app or diet tracking app like MyFitnessPal. Go grocery shopping.
5. Choose your preferred training program and research it. Read online articles, buy relevant books, download their app, sign up for their free or paid web services, and join their forums.

6. Learn the lifting movements before starting. Hire a trainer or online coach, or watch experts on YouTube to learn good form.
7. Choose a gym that has the equipment and trainer you need, or set up a gym at home.
8. Buy whatever you lack: weight scale, blender, shaker cup, protein powder, kitchen utensils, workout equipment, squat shoes, etc.
9. Take "before" pictures to easily see your progress.

Whatever thing you most dread doing next, do that first. Get it out of the way, and the rest will feel easier. You don't have to literally start everything on day one. Do it in pieces and work your way to the complete bulking program.

Quitters and Survivors

You've probably heard someone say something like, "Movies from the 90's were the best." It makes sense to look through a list of films from that decade and agree; they're all classics. The problem is, you're only seeing the good films from that era, not the stinkers like 1997's Batman and Robin.

Likewise, if you go to any beach in southern California, you'll see a lot of fit, good-looking people. You could easily assume that everyone in California is healthier. In reality, it's mostly the folks who eat right and workout that are willing to wear a bathing suit in public.

These are examples of "survivorship bias," which is our tendency as people to notice success stories (because it's all you see) while ignoring the failures. Stories of men transforming their bodies are no different. You only hear about the successes, not the more common stories of guys who worked out for a few weeks and gave up.

While this might sound like the opposite of "motivational," there's a point here. I've said a lot about how hard it is to transform your body, and it's true. Most of the guys who read this book won't fully commit to seeing the bulking program through. But there's another thing about those guys: they quit reading this book like nine chapters ago.

The point being, you're one of the survivors! Some guys bought this book, got a few chapters in, and quit. Maybe even the majority of them. If you're still reading, surely you must have something they don't. Maybe it's your drive or even a desperation to make a change. Whatever it is, it's working. Every man, deep down, wants to be swole; but you? You need it.

You no doubt have what it takes to go from scrawny to swole. The exciting part is just about to begin. Now's the time for you to have tunnel vision like you've never had it. Time to get laser focused on the next few months.

Get after it.

ABOUT THE AUTHOR

Reese Dockrey is a recreational powerlifter with a B.B.A. from the University of Texas at Arlington. When he's not busy writing or training in his garage gym in Austin, Texas, he's traveling the country as a land surveyor.

For more content and future offerings, see his website: scrawnytoswole.com.

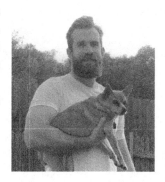

WORKS CITED

7 Body and Mind Benefits of Building Muscle. (n.d.). Retrieved July 2020, from thesource.lifetime.life: https://thesource.lifetime.life/fitness/7-body-and-mind-benefits-of-building-muscle/

Anabolic Steroid Misuse. (2018, August 30). Retrieved from nhs.uk: https://www.nhs.uk/conditions/anabolic-steroid-misuse/

Assessing Your Weight. (2020, July 1). Retrieved from cdc.gov: https://www.cdc.gov/healthyweight/assessing/index.html

Battaglia, G. (2018, December 7). *Health Risks of a Low BMI.* Retrieved from healthyeating.sfgate.com: https://healthyeating.sfgate.com/health-risks-low-bmi-5687.html

Bowerman, S. (n.d.). *Body Composition 101: Lean Body Mass and Body Fat.* Retrieved July 2020, from Discovergoodnutrition.com: https://discovergoodnutrition.com/2014/06/body-composition/

Bruusgaard et al. (2010 Aug). *Myonuclei acquired by overload exercise precede hypertrophy and are not lost on detraining.* Retrieved from researchgate.net: https://www.researchgate.net/publication/45660034_Myonuclei_acquired_by_overload_exercise_precede_hypertrophy_and_are_not_lost_on_detraining

Calories Burned in 30 Minutes for People of Three Different Weights. (2004, July). Retrieved from health.harvard.edu: https://www.health.harvard.edu/diet-and-weight-loss/calories-burned-in-30-minutes-of-leisure-and-routine-activities

Capritto, A. (2019, October 23). *Muscle pain: Is it soreness or an injury?* Retrieved from cnet.com: https://www.cnet.com/health/muscle-pain-is-it-soreness-or-an-injury/

Chavoustie, C. (2018, Oct 23). *How Big Is Your Stomach?* Retrieved from healthline.com: https://www.healthline.com/health/how-big-is-your-stomach#stomach-size

Cherney, K. (2020, June 30). *Simple Carbohydrates vs. Complex Carbohydrates.* Retrieved from healthline.com: https://www.healthline.com/health/food-nutrition/simple-carbohydrates-complex-carbohydrates

Coleman, E. (2018, December 9). *Protein and Bulking Up for Women.* Retrieved from healthyeating.sfgate.com: https://healthyeating.sfgate.com/protein-bulking-up-women-3740.html

Coleman, E. (n.d.). *Calories Needed to Gain Muscle.* Retrieved July 2020, from woman.thenest.com: https://woman.thenest.com/calories-needed-gain-muscle-5831.html

Cortes, A. (2020). *Tall Man Eating for Muscle Growth 2020.* Retrieved from cortes.site

Cortes, A. (2020). *Tall Man Training: the Strategies and Principles for Taller Men in Lifting.* Alexander Juan Antonio Cortes.

Counting Calories: Get Back to Weight-Loss Basics. (2020 July 2). Retrieved from mayoclinic.org: https://www.mayoclinic.org/healthy-lifestyle/weight-loss/in-depth/calories/art-20048065#:~:text=Because%203%2C500%20calories%20equals%20about,It%20sounds%20simple

Creicos, B. (2020, April 8). *What Is Your Body Type? Take Our Test!* Retrieved from bodybuilding.com: https://www.bodybuilding.com/fun/becker3.htm

Duquette, S. (2019, July 17). *The most attractive male body-fat percentage: is it possible to be too lean?* Retrieved from foxhoundstudio.com: https://foxhoundstudio.com/blog/the-most-attractive-male-body-fat-percentage-is-it-possible-to-be-too-lean/

Duquette, S., and Walker, M. (2020, June 23). *The Skinny Guy's Guide to Body-fat Percentage.* Retrieved from bonytobeastly.com: https://bonytobeastly.com/skinny-guys-guide-body-fat-percentage/

Duquette, S., and Walker, M. (2020, June 26). *Why is it so hard for hardgainers to gain weight?* Retrieved from bonytobeastly.com: https://bonytobeastly.com/hardgainer-weight-gain/

Ellis, E. (2020, January 20). *4 Keys to Strength Building and Muscle Mass.* Retrieved from eatright.org: https://www.eatright.org/fitness/training-and-recovery/building-muscle/strength-building-and-muscle-mass

Evans, R. (2019, January 15). *Dirty Bulking: Why You Need to Know the Dirty Truth!* Retrieved from bodybuilding.com: https://www.bodybuilding.com/content/dirty-bulking-why-you-need-to-know-the-dirty-truth.html

Feigenbaum, J. (2015, January 26). *To Be A Beast.* Retrieved from barbellmedicine.com: https://www.barbellmedicine.com/blog/584-2/

Fetters, A. (2018, March 23). *11 Benefits of Strength Training That Have Nothing to Do With Muscle Size.* Retrieved from health.usnews.com: https://health.usnews.com/wellness/fitness/articles/2018-03-23/11-benefits-of-strength-training-that-have-nothing-to-do-with-muscle-size

Fetters, A. (n.d.). *15 Negative Effects of Having a Low Body-fat Percentage.* Retrieved from mensjournal.com: https://www.mensjournal.com/health-fitness/15-negative-effects-having-low-body-fat-percentage/

Fryar, C. D. et al. (2018, September 25). *Prevalence of Underweight Among Adults Aged 20 and Over: United States, 1960–1962 Through 2015–2016.* Retrieved from cdc.gov: https://www.cdc.gov/nchs/data/hestat/underweight_adult_15_16/underweight_adult_15_16.htm#:~:text=Poor%20nutrition%20or%20underlying%20health,20%20and%20over%20are%20underweight

Garthe et al. (2010 October 7). *Effect of nutritional intervention on body composition and performance in elite athletes.* Retrieved from https://www.tandfonline.com/doi/full/10.1080/17461391.2011.643923

Garthe et al. (2011 Arp). *Effect of two different weight-loss rates on body composition and strength and power-related performance in elite athletes.* Retrieved from pubmed.ncbi.nlm.nih.gov: https://pubmed.ncbi.nlm.nih.gov/21558571/

Gelman, L. (2020 Jan 15). *Healthy Eating: 21 Food Myths You Still Think Are True.* Retrieved from thehealthy.com: https://www.thehealthy.com/food/common-food-myths/

Heffernan, A. (2020, March 14). *6 Fitness Myths That Just Won't Die.* Retrieved from menshealth.com: https://www.menshealth.com/fitness/a31491303/false-fitness-myths/

Henderson, R. (2019, July 20). *5 Reasons Why Muscles Matter, to Women and Men. New research reveals which muscles women and men consider the most attractive.* Retrieved from psychologytoday.com: https://www.psychologytoday.com/us/blog/after-service/201907/5-reasons-why-muscles-matter-women-and-men

151

How to Build Muscle: The Best Muscle-building Diet. (n.d.). Retrieved July 2020 from mensjournal.com: https://www.mensjournal.com/food-drink/how-build muscle-best-muscle-building-diet/#:~:text=According%20to%20Nate%20Miyaki%2C%20C.S.S.N.,three%20mon hs%20of%20his%20training

How to Eat Carbs for More Muscle and Less Fat. (n.d.). Retrieved July 2020, from mensjournal.com: https://www.mensjournal.com/food-drink/the-fit-5-using carbs-wisely/

Hubal et al. (2005, July). *Variability in muscle size and strength gain after unilateral resistance training.* Retrieved from researchgate.net https://www.researchgate.net/publication/7794282_Variability_in_muscle_size_a nd_strength_gain_after_unilateral_resistance_training

Hyson, S. (n.d.). *Here's Why You Don't Need to Spike Your Insulin After a Workout.* Retrieved July 2020, from mensjournal.com https://www.mensjournal.com/food-drink/heres-why-you-dont-need-spike-your-insulin-after-workout/

Iliades, C. (2019, May 13). *7 Ways Strength Training Boosts your Health and Fitness.* Retrieved from everydayhealth.com https://www.everydayhealth.com/fitness/add-strength-training-to-your-workout.aspx

Iraki et al. (2019 June 26). *Nutrition Recommendations for Bodybuilders in the Off Season: A Narrative Review.* Retrieved from https://www.ncbi.nlm.nih.gov/pmc/articles/PMC6680710/

John, D. (2009). *Never Let Go: A Philosophy of Lifting, Living and Learning.* On Target Publications.

John, D. (2020). *Mass Made Simple: A Six-Week Journey into Bulking.* On Target Publications, LLC.

Kamb, S. (2020, January 1). *How Fast Can I Build Muscle Naturally? A Step-By-Step Buide to Building Muscle Quickly.* Retrieved from nerdfitness.com https://www.nerdfitness.com/blog/how-fast-can-i-build-muscle-naturally/

Kamb, S. (2020, January 1). *How Many Sets and Reps Should I Do? (Building The Correct Workout Plan).* Retrieved from nerdfitness.com https://www.nerdfitness.com/blog/the-correct-number-of-reps-per-set-in-the-gym/

Klepchukova, A. (2020, April 25). *10 Fitness Myths vs. Truth.* Retrieved from flo.health: https://flo.health/menstrual-cycle/lifestyle/fitness-and-exercise/10-fitness-myths-vs-truth

Kresser, C. (2019, February 19). *How Industrial Seed Oils Are Making Us Sick.* Retrieved from chriskresser.com: https://chriskresser.com/how-industrial-seed-oils-are-making-us-sick/

Lee, S. (2015, July 8). *What the Heck "Newbie Gains" Are, and What to Do Afterward.* Retrieved from vitals.lifehacker.com: https://vitals.lifehacker.com/what-the-heck-newbie-gains-are-and-what-to-do-afterw-1716332727

Legge, A. (n.d.). *How Fast Can You Lose Fat Without Losing Muscle? (According to Science).* Retrieved July 2020, from legionathletics.com: https://legionathletics.com/lose-fat-fast/

Legge, A. (n.d.). *How Fast You Lose Muscle When You Stop Working Out.* Retrieved July 2020, from legionathletics.com: https://legionathletics.com/how-fast-you-lose-muscle-when-you-stop-working-out/#how-fast-will-you-lose-muscle-if-you-stop-working-out

Levine et al. (2000, Dec). *Energy Expenditure of Nonexercise Activity.* Retrieved from pubmed.ncbi.nlm.nih.gov: https://pubmed.ncbi.nlm.nih.gov/11101470/

MacDonald, Ann. (2010, October 19). *Why Eating Slowly May Help You Feel Full Faster.* Retrieved from health.harvard.edu: https://www.health.harvard.edu/blog/why-eating-slowly-may-help-you-feel-full-faster-20101019605

Matthews, M. (n.d.). *Are Compound Exercises Better Than Isolation Exercises?* Retrieved July 2020, from legionathletics.com: https://legionathletics.com/compound-exercises/#what-is-a-compound-exercise

Matthews, M. (n.d.). *Here's How Much Muscle You Can Really Gain Naturally (with a Calculator).* Retrieved from legionathletics.com: https://legionathletics.com/how-to-build-muscle-naturally/

Matthews, M. (n.d.). *How Dangerous Is Weightlifting? What 20 Studies Have to Say.* Retrieved July 2020, from legionathletics.com: https://legionathletics.com/is-weightlifting-dangerous/

Matthews, M. (n.d.). *How to Calculate Your Body Fat Percentage Easily & Accurately (With a Calculator).* Retrieved July 2020, from legionathletics.com: https://legionathletics.com/how-to-calculate-body-fat/#whats-a-healthy-body-fat-percentage-for-men-and-women

Matthews, M. (n.d.). *How to Maintain Muscle and Strength with Minimal Exercise.* Retrieved from legionathletics.com: https://legionathletics.com/maintain-muscle-and-strength/

Matthews, M. (n.d.). *Muscle Memory Is Real and Here's How It Helps You Build Muscle Fast.* Retrieved from legionathletics.com: https://legionathletics.com/muscle-memory/

McDonald, L. (2009, June 19). *Four Models for Genetic Muscular Potential.* Retrieved from bodyrecomposition.com: https://bodyrecomposition.com/muscle-gain/genetic-muscular-potential

McGrath, B. (2018, July 24). *4 Tips To Help Train Your Brain For Massive Gains: Mind Muscle Connection!* Retrieved from bodybuilding.com: https://www.bodybuilding.com/content/4-tips-to-help-train-your-brain-massive-gains-mind-muscle-connection.html

McKay, B. (2020, July 24). *How to Gain Weight.* Retrieved from artofmanliness.com: https://www.artofmanliness.com/articles/how-to-gain-weight/

McKay, B. M. (2020, July 13). *The Herschel Walker Workout.* Retrieved from artofmanliness.com: https://www.artofmanliness.com/articles/the-herschel-walker-workout/

Metabolism and weight loss: How you burn calories. (2017, August 30). Retrieved from mayoclinic.org: https://www.mayoclinic.org/healthy-lifestyle/weight-loss/in-depth/metabolism/art-20046508

Nippard, J. (2020 May 31). *How to Re-Build Muscle After A Training Break.* Retrieved from youtube.com: https://www.youtube.com/watch?v=LiyDfoUkbdo&app=desktop&t=7s

Nuckols, Greg. (2017 January 3). *Data-Based Muscle, Strength, and Fat-Loss Targets to Set Realistic Training Goals.* Retrieved from https://www.strongerbyscience.com/realistic-training-goals/

Obesity and Overweight. (2016, June 13). Retrieved from cdc.gov: https://www.cdc.gov/nchs/fastats/obesity-overweight.htm

Park, M. (2010, November 8). *Twinkie Diet Helps Nutrition Professor Lose 27 Pounds.* Retrieved from cnn.com: http://www.cnn.com/2010/HEALTH/11/08/twinkie.diet.professor/index.html

Pendick, D. (2015, June 18). *How Much Protein Do You Need Every Day?* Retrieved from health.harvard.edu: https://www.health.harvard.edu/blog/how-much-protein-do-you-need-every-day-201506188096

Physiology of Strength Training: Stress, Recovery, Adaptation. (n.d.). Retrieved July 2020, from barbell-logic.com: https://barbell-logic.com/physiology-of-strength-training/

Preiato, D. (2020, April 8). *Where Does Fat Go When You Lose Weight?* Retrieved from healthline.com: https://www.healthline.com/nutrition/where-does-fat-go-when-you-lose-weight#1

r/gainit We're All Gonna Make It! (n.d.). Retrieved July 2020, from reddit.com: https://www.reddit.com/r/gainit/

Reid, F. (n.d.). *Sarcoplasmic & Myofibrillar Hypertrophy | What Is It?* Retrieved July 2020, from myprotein.com: https://www.myprotein.com/thezone/training/sarcoplasmic-myofibrillar-hypertrophy-what-is-it/

Ribeiro et al. (2019, February). *Effects of Different Dietary Energy Intake Following Resistance Training on Muscle Mass and Body Fat in Bodybuilders: A Pilot Study.* Retrieved from https://www.researchgate.net/publication/331071618_Effects_of_Different_Dietary_Energy_Intake_Following_Resistance_Training_on_Muscle_Mass_and_Body_Fat_in_Bodybuilders_A_Pilot_Study

Rippetoe, M. (2010, May 7). *A Clarification.* Retrieved from startingstrength.com: https://startingstrength.com/article/a_clarification

Rippetoe, M. (2015, December 30). *The First Three Questions.* Retrieved from startingstrength.com: https://startingstrength.com/article/the_first_three_questions

Rippetoe, M. (2017, January 13). *Maybe You Should GAIN Weight.* Retrieved from startingstrength.com: https://startingstrength.com/article/maybe-you-should-gain-weight

Rippetoe, M. (2017). *Starting Strength: Basic Barbell Training* (3 ed.). The Aasgaard Company.

Rodal, R. (2018, July 18). *5 Weight Lifting Injuries That Are Far Too Common.* Retrieved from tigerfitness.com: https://www.tigerfitness.com/blogs/workouts/5-weight-lifting-injuries

Satrazemis, E. (2019 March 14). *How Many Calories Should I Eat to Gain Weight?* Retrieved from trifectanutrition.com: https://www.trifectanutrition.com/blog/how-many-calories-should-i-eat-to-gain-weight

Schultz, R. (n.d.). *The Real Danger of Too Much Protein.* Retrieved July 2020, from mensjournal.com: https://www.mensjournal.com/food-drink/real-danger-too-much-protein/. Accessed 31 July 2020

Seaborne et al. (2018 Jan 30). *Human Skeletal Muscle Possesses an Epigenetic Memory of Hypertrophy.* Retrieved from nature.com: https://www.nature.com/articles/s41598-018-20287-3

Shugart, Chris. (2004 Oct 21). *All Muscle, No Iron: An Interview with Coach Christopher Sommer.* Retrieved from t-nation.com: https://www.t-nation.com/training/all-muscle-no-iron

Stress and Sleep. (2013) Retrieved from apa.org: https://www.apa.org/news/press/releases/stress/2013/sleep

Tavel, R. (2018 Nov 21). *How You Can Use Hypertrophy to Grow Your Muscles.* Retrieved from menshealth.com: https://www.menshealth.com/fitness/a25252586/muscle-hypertrophy/

The Truth About Fats: the Good, the Bad, and the In-betweens. (2019, December 11). Retrieved from health.harvard.edu: https://www.health.harvard.edu/staying-healthy/the-truth-about-fats-bad-and-good

Thieme, T. (2019, June 10). *Why You Really Want to Focus on Your Muscle Pump.* Retrieved from menshealth.com: https://www.menshealth.com/fitness/a19520337/muscle-pump-builds-size-and-strength/

Weatherspoon, D. (2019, June 10). *All About Testosterone in Women.* Retrieved from healthline.com: https://www.healthline.com/health/womens-health/do-women-have-testosterone

Weight training appears key to controlling belly fat. (2014, December 22). Retrieved from hsph.harvard.edu: https://www.hsph.harvard.edu/news/press-releases/weight-training-appears-key-to-controlling-belly-fat/

Your Body Type- Ectomorph, Mesomorph or Endomorph? (n.d.). Retrieved July 2020, from muscleandstrength.com: https://www.muscleandstrength.com/articles/body-types-ectomorph-mesomorph-endomorph.html

Zeratsky, K. (2019, March 3). *What's an Easy Way to See How Much Fat I Eat Each Day?* Retrieved from mayoclinic.org: https://www.mayoclinic.org/healthy-lifestyle/nutrition-and-healthy-eating/expert-answers/fat-grams/faq-20058496

Made in the USA
Las Vegas, NV
23 December 2023

83467391R00095